author

i A. Kalender, born in 1949, studied physics and medical physics in
n, Germany, and at the University of Wisconsin, Madison, Wisconsin,
ve for 16 years in CT research & development at the Siemens Medical
ineering Group in Erlangen, Germany. Professor and chairman of the
itute of Medical Physics (IMP) at the University Erlangen-Nuremberg
e 1995.

obtain further and topical information on the author or further projects
work, especially related to new developments in CT, please visit our
rnet Homepage www.imp.uni-erlangen.de at any time.

Computed Tom

Computed Tomography

Fundamentals, System Technology,
Image Quality, Applications

Willi A. Kalender

Publicis MCD Verlag

Die Deutsche Bibliothek – CIP-Cataloguing-in-Publication-Data
A catalogue record for this publication is available from Die Deutsche Bibliothek

ISBN 3-89578-081-2

Editor: Publicis MCD Werbeagentur GmbH, Munich
Publisher: Publicis MCD Verlag
© 2000 by Publicis MCD Werbeagentur GmbH, Munich

Printed in Germany

Preface

X-ray computed tomography (CT) brought slice imaging into wide use for the first time and represented its breakthrough. Today, CT is an essential part of radiological diagnostics and can be seen as a mature and clinically accepted procedure. It has supplemented or replaced classical x-ray imaging in many areas.

A rapid technical development phase in the seventies was followed by an uneventful phase with no essential highlights in the eighties. This was partly caused by the expectation that the importance of CT would decrease successively due to the introduction of magnetic resonance (MR) tomography. Contrary to these expectations, CT is in a phase of rapid technical development and again broadening its application spectrum. The development of spiral CT and the transition from scanning single slices to the rapid scanning of complete volumes has made CT attractive again and has led to decisive developments in technical and in clinical perspectives. The introduction of multi-row detector systems and scan times in the subsecond range currently constitute the high point of these developments.

The present book is intended to describe technical and physical aspects of computed tomography, from sequential single-slice scanning to volume scanning by multi-slice spiral CT (MSCT). The fundamentals of CT are described in detail in the first chapter for "CT novices" in an illustrative manner. Readers familiar with this material may skip this chapter or refresh their knowledge by following the figures. Mathematical principles which are not required for the understanding of the following chapters are summarized as an appendix in chapter 9.

In addition to the necessary CT basics, the most recent developments and future-oriented considerations are presented in depth in chapters 2 to 4. Chapter 2 is dedicated to technical concepts in CT and the corresponding apparatus and scan modes, chapter 3 to spiral CT and chapter 4 to image quality considerations. The focus is always on problems relevant to the user of CT equipment. In particular, this includes the potential and the results of the new multi-row detector systems and the corresponding scan and reconstruction options, which have not been covered in detail in any textbook up to now. The routine availability of high isotropic resolution in all three dimensions is the eminent result.

In view of the importance of radiation protection, both in principle and with respect to the high topical importance in Europe, questions regarding dose and possibilities for patient dose reduction are discussed separately in depth in chapter 5. The possibilities for dose reduction are emphasized, and new concepts such as tube current modulation and an automatic exposure control for CT are explained. Such measures to reduce dose and to offer information on actual organ dose values should free CT from the generally held misconception of being a "high dose modality". Effective dose values for typical CT examinations are on the order of the natural background radiation per year.

2D and 3D approaches to display, to visualize and to diagnose CT images are explained in chapter 6. Interactive approaches continuously gaining importance for the data volumes encountered today are also illustrated by examples and interactive exercises on the CD-ROM. In chapter 7, some fundamental remarks on and clinical examples for special applications follow with CT imaging of the heart, as one of the potentially most future-prone new applications being described in detail. Chapter 8 offers a brief assessment of the prospects for future developments in CT.

The material in this book is supported by image examples, video clips and the possibility of interactive exercises for image display and processing on the enclosed CD-ROM. The respective supplements are indicated in the text. Example images for most body regions and some volume data sets can be loaded, windowed, magnified and viewed interactively. Above all for "novices" – such as students or colleagues working in other fields who do not have access to a CT scanner or to CT data – this offers the possibility to familiarize themselves with results of CT imaging under realistic conditions. The CD-ROM also includes all figures of this book in digital form, i.e. in full quality. To appreciate all details in some of the clinical examples, it may be of help to look them up on the CD-ROM.

The book is addressed to a wide interdisciplinary readership in an effort to explain both the fundamentals and applications of CT. Consequently, the focus is on physics and technology, whereas radiological aspects are addressed only marginally. There is no requirement for special prior knowledge. With respect to detail problems or questions, relevant literature is referenced. Important CT terms are assembled in the glossary and defined briefly. Whether the stated goals have been achieved remains open to the judgement of the reader. The author is open to suggestions, comments and criticism at any time.

Acknowledgements

It is not possible to mention all those by name who have contributed directly or indirectly to the generation of all the material in and to the completion of this book. This would have to include the many colleagues and partners in cooperations who supported me during two decades of work in CT development and who were available for many discussions.

All newer CT images in this book and on the CD-ROM have been generated on the SOMATOM Volume Zoom (VZ) which was provided to the Institute of Medical Physics (IMP) in August 1998 by the Siemens Medical Engineering Group for experimental and clinical work. I would like to explicitly acknowledge this support and the willingness of many colleagues at Siemens to cooperate on numerous projects. The results, e.g. on image quality assessment, dose reduction and CT imaging of the heart, speak for the success of this cooperation.

Many colleagues from the Institute of Radiology of the University of Erlangen, under the direction of Werner Bautz, have been excellent partners in the most recent CT projects. I would like to thank especially Ulrich Baum and Michael Lell for selecting and providing the clinical CT images.

I am particularly grateful to the coworkers at my own institute who have supported me during project "CT – the book" in relaxed manner, with constructive criticism and tireless efforts: thanks are due to Daniel Schwartz (figures), Marie-Theres Reim (text layout), Theo Fuchs, Marc Kachelrieß, Bernhard Schmidt, Markus Blank and Stefan Ulzheimer. Should you be interested in learning about the persons behind these names, you can find further information under www.imp.uni-erlangen.de/team.

I am most grateful of all to Marlene, who also tolerated and supported the project "CT – the book" in relaxed manner as usual and with valuable efforts to turn my English into English. Should you be interested in further information about the person behind this name, this is only available privately.

Erlangen, July 2000   Willi A. Kalender

Table of Contents

Historical Overview

"If we give free rein to our fantasy and imagine perfecting the new photographic process with the aid of Crookes' tube until one part of the soft-tissue structures of the human body remains transparent and a layer located underneath can be imaged on the plate, this would be of invaluable assistance in diagnosing innumerable diseases not directly associated with bone structures"

Translation of an excerpt from the
'Frankfurter Zeitung', January 7, 1896.

Ideas and concepts for tomographic imaging with x-rays were developed early. The unknown author of the above article appearing in the feature supplement of the 'Frankfurter Zeitung' expressed truly prophetic thoughts only a few days after the first reports were published on Roentgen's discovery of X-rays and prior to their first medical use. We do not know what the author had in mind when he conceived the possibility of displaying "... the soft tissue structures ... and a layer located underneath ...". It was certainly not computed tomography as we know it today. Perhaps he wished to obtain a view similar to that with an anatomical preparation after superimposed layers of tissue have been removed. His assessment that ".... this would be of invaluable assistance in diagnosing innumerable diseases not directly associated with bone structures" was in any case correct. One should, however, avoid over-interpretation of this quotation; the development of tomography, modern methods of reconstructing digital images, and today's powerful computers were as yet undreamed of.

Computed tomography (CT) first became feasible with the development of modern computer technology in the sixties, but some of the ideas on which it is based can be traced back to the first half of this century. In 1917 the Bohemian mathematician J.H. Radon [Radon, 1917] proved in a research paper of fundamental importance that the distribution of a material or material property in an object layer can be calculated if the integral values along any number of lines passing through the same layer are known. The first applications of this theory were developed for radioastronomy by Bracewell in 1956 [Bracewell, 1956], but they met with little response and were not exploited for medical purposes.

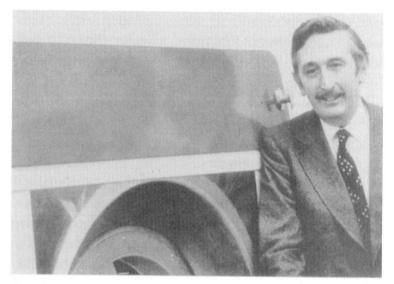

Figure 1
Godfrey N. Hounsfield, the English engineer who developed the first CT scanner and received the Nobel Prize in medicine in 1979 together with the physicist A.M. Cormack.

The first experiments on medical applications of this type of reconstructive tomography were carried out by the physicist A.M. Cormack, who worked on improving radiotherapy planning at Groote Schuur Hospital, Cape Town, South Africa. Between 1957 and 1963, and without knowledge of previous studies, he developed a method of calculating radiation absorption distributions in the human body based on transmission measurements [Cormack, 1963]. He postulated for radiological applications that it must be possible to display even the most minute absorption differences, i.e. different soft-tissue structures. However, he never had occasion to put his theory into practice and first learned of Radon's work much later, a fact that he regretted by stating that earlier access to this knowledge would have saved him a lot of work. While familiarizing himself with Radon's work, Cormack discovered that Radon had himself been unaware of even earlier work on the subject by the Dutch physicist H. A. Lorentz, who had already proposed a solution of the mathematical problem for the 3D case in 1905 [Cormack, 1992].

A successful practical implementation of this theory was first achieved in 1972 by the English engineer G.N. Hounsfield, who is now generally recognized as the inventor of computed tomography [Hounsfield, 1973]. Like his predecessors, Hounsfield worked without knowledge of the above-mentioned earlier findings. His success took the entire medical world by surprise, and he achieved his remarkable breakthrough neither at a renowned university nor with a leading manufacturer of radiological equip-

Table 1 Historical overview: the development of CT

1895	W.C. Roentgen discovers 'a new kind of rays', later referred to as 'X-rays' or 'roentgen rays' in his honor.
1917	J. H. Radon develops the mathematical foundation for reconstructing cross-sectional images from transmission measurements [Radon, 1917].
1963	A.M. Cormack describes a technique for calculating the absorption distribution in the human body [Cormack, 1963].
1972	G.N. Hounsfield and J. Ambrose conduct the first clinical CT examinations [Hounsfield, 1973].
1974	60 clinical CT installations (head scanners)
1975	First whole-body CT scanner in clinical use.
1979	Hounsfield and Cormack awarded the Nobel Prize.
1989	W.A. Kalender and P. Vock conduct the first clinical examinations with spiral CT [Kalender, 1989; Kalender, 1990b].
1998	Introduction of multi-slice detector systems
2000	approx. 30,000 clinical CT installations (whole body scanners)

ment, but with the British firm EMI Ltd. His invention gave EMI, which had until then manufactured only records and electronic components, a monopoly in the CT market that lasted for 2 years, and the terms 'EMI Scanner' and 'CT Scanner' became almost synonymous. In 1974 Siemens became the first traditional manufacturer of radiological equipment to market a head CT Scanner, after which many other companies quickly followed suit. A boom followed, reaching its peak in the late seventies with 18 companies offering CT equipment. Most of these, including EMI, have withdrawn from the market by now.

The first clinical CT images were produced at the Atkinson Morley Hospital in London in 1972. The very first patient examination performed with CT offered convincing proof of the effectiveness of the method by detecting a cystic frontal lobe tumor. CT was immediately and enthusiastically welcomed by the medical community, and has often been referred to as the most important invention in diagnostic radiology since the discovery of X-rays; its later development only confirmed these early expectations. Computed tomography has become a very important factor in radiological diagnosis. While only 60 EMI scanners had been installed by 1974, there were more than 10,000 devices in use in 1980, including a high number of head scanners. In 1979 Hounsfield and Cormack, an engineer and a physicist, were awarded the Nobel Prize for medicine in recognition of their outstanding achievements.

At this point, the development seemed to have reached its peak, and the eighties saw scarcely any technological progress. Only the introduction of spiral CT [Kalender, 1990b] and the following developments in x-ray, detector and scanner technology have led to a renewal of interest in clinical applications. For the year 2000, the number of clinical installations in operation is estimated to be approx. 30,000; almost exclusively whole body scanners. The upward trend is unbroken for the time being, and the position of CT is consolidated despite further developments in other radiological methods.

1 Principles of Computed Tomography

1.1 General Considerations on Slice Imaging

CT was the first widely used radiological imaging modality which exclusively provided computed digital images instead of the well known directly acquired analog images. And it offered images of single discrete slices instead of superposition images of complete body sections. The two characteristics "digital" and "volume representation by single slices", which were new at the time, are in the meantime familiar and are also associated with other slice imaging modalities such as ultrasound, magnetic resonance tomography (MRT) and positron emission tomography (PET). Are there any limitations or disadvantages associated with these two characteristics? What advantages do they offer? In the section following below a short discussion of the principal considerations is offered for the interested reader. It will be shown that the characteristics "digital" and "volume representation by single slices" are hardly noticeable these days and that contrast which is defined locally for slice images constitutes the decisive principal difference compared with conventional x-ray imaging. Readers familiar with medical imaging in general and with CT may possibly glance over the figures only or immediately continue with chapter 1.2 or chapter 2, respectively.

1.1.1 Computed Tomography – a Digital Modality

We have been familiar with radiographs, i.e. imaging of parts of the human body by means of x-rays and film, for about a century now. Anatomy is presented on the analog medium film as a continuum with nearly arbitrary fine transitions, similar in this respect to photographic pictures on film. The human eye does not recognize any steps in intensity or discrete picture elements. Intuitively one assumes that arbitrarily fine gradations of gray levels and continuous transitions for contours are given. The situation is similar to the hearing process: the human ear subjectively perceives a continuous frequency spectrum when listening to music or arbitrary natural sounds. In both cases – in visual and in auditory perception – analog recordings are classified as "arbitrarily fine", while digital is often associated with "coarse or discrete sampling".

Today we have come to recognize and accept – and with respect to the example of audio records, even most admirers of good old analog records do so as well – that the same high recording and perception quality can be

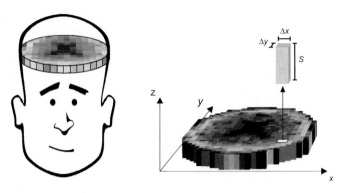

Figure 1.1
Computed tomography – perception in slices. CT provides transverse slice images of the human body in digital form. A coordinate system then results which basically conforms to the anatomical main axes and planes.

made available with digital media. For CT, this was definitely not the case in the early days.

For an understanding of computed tomography it may be helpful to view the human body as built up of a finite number of discrete slices and volume elements. Each single scan aims to determine the composition of one transverse cross-section. This respective slice or section can be imagined in turn as composed of discrete cubic volume elements (figure 1.1). The value attached to each volume element is displayed in one picture element of the digital image matrix. For volume elements we often use the acronym "voxel", and for picture elements the term "pixel".

In principle, a slice image can be generated in arbitrary orientation. For CT as well as PET, however, mostly a transverse plane which is here labeled as the x/y-plane is scanned directly. The z-axis, oriented perpendicular to the scan and image plane, is thereby aligned along the axis of rotation of the scanning system and thus approximately parallel to the body's longitudinal axis (figure 1.1). Sagittal body sections are approximated by y/z-planes, and coronal sections by x/z-planes.

The edge lengths of a voxel in this coordinate system are determined by the pixel size, resulting from the selected matrix size and field of view (see section 4.1.3.2), and the slice thickness S. For coarse matrices, a chessboard-like impression may result. This was in fact the case for early CT images which were reconstructed, fully adequate for the low spatial resoluton at that time, with an 80 × 80 matrix (figure 1.2a). The impression is disturbing, however; the quality of such a digital image is obviously still limited. Multiplanar representations in planes perpendicular to the scan plane also exhibit a coarse appearance depending on the slice thickness

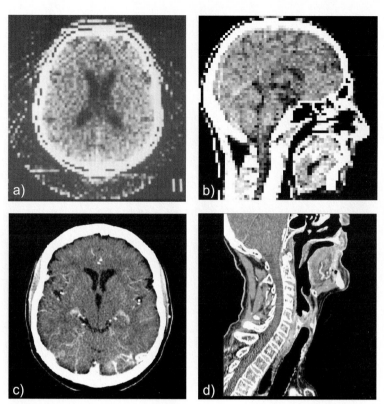

Figure 1.2
Analog or digital images? Continuous imaging of anatomy or scanning of single slices? In early CT images, here a brain scan produced in 1974 with an 80 × 80 image matrix **(a)**, the computed discrete picture elements are clearly visible, just as the steps in the secondary reconstructions generated from single scans taken with a spacing of 13 mm **(b)**. Volume scans obtained in spiral scanning mode and reconstruction of matrices with 1024 × 1024 picture elements **(c)** cannot be discerned from analog images anymore; they can also be viewed in the third dimension quasi-continuously **(d)**.

(figure 1.2b). These limitations in image quality are not of a fundamental nature; they result from limitations in the techniques used.

The chapters following below will further illustrate that the question "analog or digital?" does not bear high relevance for CT imaging anymore, as was the case in the early days of CT (figure 1.2a,b). Matrix sizes and spatial resolution for the imaged slice have reached values which hardly allow a differentiation – no matter whether the image has been generated quasi in an analog manner or built up from discrete picture elements (figure 1.2c). The image remains digital in nature of course; pixels can be made visible by high magnification of any arbitrary image. This can be verified by a simple exercise using the Magnify function in the evaluation software on the enclosed CD-ROM.

Only for the third dimension, along the z-axis in our coordinate system, can the effects of low spatial resolution and large slice thickness often still be recognized. Choosing thin slice widths and overlapping image reconstruction for spiral CT or multi-slice spiral CT scans meanwhile provides the quality of analog images to a good approximation (figure 1.2d). Digital images with their computed discrete picture elements, which have come into broad use in radiology through CT, do not entail any disadvantages.

1.1.2   Why do Slice Images offer Higher Contrast?

Conventional film radiography offered a valuable non-invasive means of diagnosis for many decades. Its limitations were and are severe, however; we are increasingly less aware of these due to the availability of alternative procedures. Imaging the brain by radiographs, for example, yields insufficient results in most cases. Roentgenologists tried to solve this dilemma by various measures, for example by using contrast media such as air in pneumoencephalography. In spite of the high efforts and the great discomfort to the patient these procedures only yielded very limited additional information. Computed tomography for the first time offered the possibility to image brain structures in diagnostic quality with high contrast (figure 1.3). How is this achieved? Several radiological text books have offered the explanation that the high contrast of CT images is due to the higher dose. This explanation is wrong. Although both radiography and CT use x-rays, CT images display a quantity different from that in radiographs.

The principle of radiography is to record the radiation which is emitted from the focus of an x-ray tube and attenuated by the object to be examined with a detector, traditionally by film. Thus, a conventional radiograph presents the modulated distribution of radiation intensity and always offers a superposition image: all structures along the rays from x-ray focus to detector, i.e. all volume elements passed by any ray, contribute to the attenuation of the radiation intensity. Each picture element displays the sum of all contributions to attenuation or, mathematically speaking, the integral of the attenuation components along a line. We will return to these

Figure 1.3 ▶
Why does CT offer higher contrast?
a) CT images display the attenuation resulting from each volume element directly assigned to the respective single picture element. Accordingly, contrast in CT is defined by local differences in attenuation and the lesion is easily recognized.
b) Projection images, in this case the conventional radiograph of the skull, render the sum of all signal contributions along a ray from the x-ray source to each picture element. In such a superposition image, only structures can be recognized which exhibit very high differences in attenuation with respect to their surroundings.
c) The high contrast offered by CT images – here only illustrated by way of numbers – is due to the imaging principle and not due to radiation dose or scan parameters.

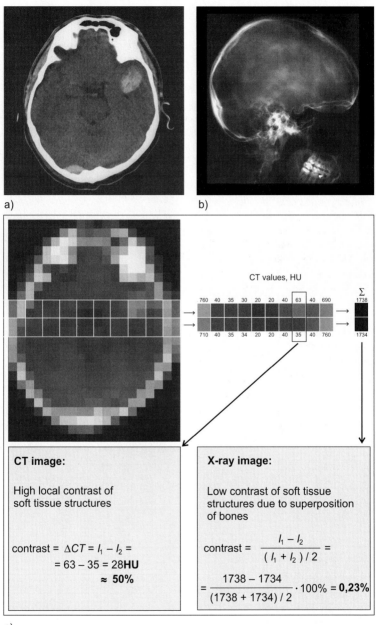

a)

b)

CT values, HU

760	40	35	30	20	20	40	63	40	690

Σ 1738

710	40	35	34	20	20	40	35	40	760

1734

CT image:

High local contrast of
soft tissue structures

contrast = $\Delta CT = I_1 - I_2 =$
$= 63 - 35 = 28\textbf{HU}$
$\approx \textbf{50\%}$

X-ray image:

Low contrast of soft tissue
structures due to superposition
of bones

contrast = $\dfrac{I_1 - I_2}{(I_1 + I_2)/2} =$

$= \dfrac{1738 - 1734}{(1738 + 1734)/2} \cdot 100\% = \textbf{0,23\%}$

c)

"line integrals" again when discussing the principle of computed tomography in the next section.

Image contrast is defined by the difference in intensity of two neighboring picture elements or regions. This definition holds true in the same way for conventional radiographs and for CT images. Contrast in radiographs is dominated by structures with high attenuation such as bone and contrast media or by differences in object thickness. Contributions from structures with low attenuation, typically soft tissue structures, are thereby completely hidden in most practical cases. This fundamental problem in conventional imaging cannot be eliminated. Even the introduction of improved detector systems or digital data processing will not alter the situation.

For slice images contrast is given directly by the attenuation values of neighboring volume elements or subvolumes and not by line integrals representing a path through the complete object. Contrast is determined locally by the composition of the tissues, while neighboring or super-imposed structures have no or only very little influence. Arbitrarily small differences in the density or the composition of tissues can therefore be rendered with sufficient contrast as a matter of principle. This statement is true for all slice imaging modalities. This decisive advantage of slice imaging, illustrated in an examplary fashion in figure 1.3c, led to the immediate breakthrough of CT with its introduction in the year 1972.

1.2   Basic Principles of CT

In general terms, the principle of computed tomography consists of measuring the spatial distribution of a physical quantity to be examined from different directions and to compute superposition free images from these data. This abstract principle will be illustrated for sequential CT, i.e. the scanning of single slices, in an illustrative way by answering the questions following below. The underlying mathematical foundations will be left out as much as possible. A short description of these is offered in chapter 9.2; detailed elaborations are found in the literature, for example in [Brooks, 1976; Scudder, 1978; Morneburg, 1995].

1.2.1   What do we Measure in CT?

For survey radiographs, the relative distribution of the x-ray intensity is recorded; i.e. for classical radiographs only the gray value pattern is utilized to derive a diagnosis. In CT, the intensity of x-rays is also recorded behind the object. In addition to the intensity I attenuated by the object, the primary intensity I_0 has to be measured in CT to calculate the attenuation value along each ray from source to detector. The respective formula and some simple cases are illustrated in figure 1.4.

The simplest case is given by a measurement of a homogeneous object with monochromatic radiation (figure 1.4, case 1); this case does not necessarily demand tomographic imaging, but it is familiar to us from many different measurement procedures. The intensity falls off exponentially with absorber thickness. Attenuation, defined as the natural logarithm of the ratio of primary intensity to attenuated intensity, is given in this case in a simple manner as the product of the linear attenuation coefficient μ and the absorber thickness d. If the absorber thickness is known μ can be determined directly. The distribution of μ along the ray path remains unknown, however.

Case 2 in figure 1.4, representing a simple inhomogeneous object, is of greater interest. The contribution to total attenuation resulting from each ray path interval depends on the local value of the attenuation coefficient μ_i. Summation over the path intervals, even for simply structured objects, has to be carried out in general with small increments d_i and therefore can be expressed as the integral over μ along the ray path. CT consists of measuring many such line integrals exactly. Radon showed in his early work [Radon, 1917] that the two-dimensional distribution of an object characteristic can be determined exactly if an infinite number of line integrals is given. A finite number of measurements of the distribution of the attenuation coefficient $\mu(x,y)$ is sufficient to compute an image to a good approximation. A single measurement only, as given in projection radiography, will not allow us to solve for μ_i in case 2 or for the distribution $\mu(x,y)$ in general.

Before explaining how the measurement has to be carried out and how an image can be computed it must be said that the linear attenuation coefficient may depend strongly on energy. In measuring intensities – and this is done automatically in today's CT systems – we also integrate over all energy intervals as illustrated for case 3 of figure 1.4. The dependence on energy may yield problems, above all beam hardening effects, which will be discussed in chapter 4. However, this can also be used in dual energy methods for material-selective measurements. If we also consider a potential dependence of attenuation on time, the measured quantity in CT, the linear coefficient is given as $\mu(x,y,z,E,t)$. A dependence of μ on time can be generated by the administration of contrast media or be given by physiology, for example in lung tissue as a function of inspiratory volume. In the following sections we will focus on the simple case of measuring and computing $\mu(x,y)$ only for a given slice position z.

1.2.2 How do we Measure an Object in CT?

To be able to compute an image in acceptable quality following Radon's theory, a sufficiently high number of attenuation integrals or projection values have to be recorded. It is necessary to carry out measurements in all

Case 1: homogeneous object, monochromatic radiation

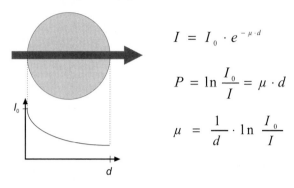

$$I = I_0 \cdot e^{-\mu \cdot d}$$

$$P = \ln \frac{I_0}{I} = \mu \cdot d$$

$$\mu = \frac{1}{d} \cdot \ln \frac{I_0}{I}$$

Case 2: inhomogeneous object, monochromatic radiation

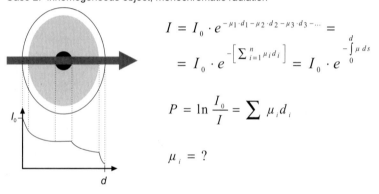

$$I = I_0 \cdot e^{-\mu_1 \cdot d_1 - \mu_2 \cdot d_2 - \mu_3 \cdot d_3 - \dots} =$$

$$= I_0 \cdot e^{-\left[\sum_{i=1}^{n} \mu_i d_i \right]} = I_0 \cdot e^{-\int_0^d \mu \, ds}$$

$$P = \ln \frac{I_0}{I} = \sum \mu_i d_i$$

$$\mu_i = ?$$

Case 3: inhomogeneous object, polychromatic radiation

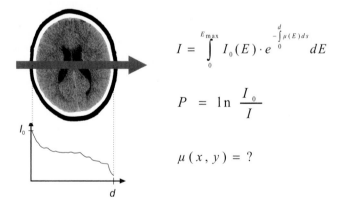

$$I = \int_0^{E_{max}} I_0(E) \cdot e^{-\int_0^d \mu(E) \, ds} \, dE$$

$$P = \ln \frac{I_0}{I}$$

$$\mu(x, y) = ?$$

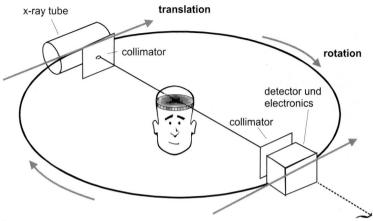

Figure 1.5
How do we measure an object in CT?
In the simplest case x-ray intensities and therefore object attenuation will be measured
with a pencil beam for many different angular positions.

directions, i.e. at least over an angular range of 180°, and to determine
many narrowly spaced data points for each projection.

A simple measurement setup fulfilling this purpose is sketched in figure
1.5. A radiation source with adequate collimation emits a pencil beam and
the intensity, attenuated by the object, is registered by the detector placed
opposite. For a given angular position, this setup of radiation source and
detector is moved linearly (translation), and the intensity is measured either
at single discrete points or continuously. This results in an intensity profile
recorded for parallel rays. By determining the ratios of the primary intensity recorded in the periphery and the attenuated intensities recorded
behind the object and taking their logarithms, an attenuation profile results
which is generally termed a projection. Projections are measured successively for successive angular positions. The complete set of projections,
here determined in parallel ray geometry over 180°, is then transferred to
the data processing unit. Exactly this procedure was used in the first clinical CT scanners, with 180 projections taken in 1° angular intervals (step-
wise rotation) with 160 data points measured per projection.

CT scanners today measure typically in fan-beam geometry over an angular range of 360°. The extension to 360° resulted from several considera-

◀ **Figure 1.4**
What do we measure in CT? The intensity I of radiation. The attenuation value, i.e. the
projection value P, results and thus, in the simplest case, the attenuation coefficient μ (case
1). For inhomogeneous objects tomographic imaging is necessary to determine the distribution $\mu(x,y)$.

tions, initially focussing on image quality and better data sampling. By proper geometrical alignment of the detector, the quarter detector offset, overlapping sampling is achieved (s. section 2.2.1). Practical considerations also demand 360° scanning; for spiral CT in particular, this is a prerequisite. Modern CT scanners typically measure 800–1,500 projections with 600–1,200 data points per projection.

1.2.3 How do we Compute a CT Image?

Information on the as yet unknown distribution $\mu(x,y)$ of attenuation coefficients is only given in form of a set of projection values, which is also termed the "Radon transform" of the image. An inverse transformation has to be carried out to determine $\mu(x,y)$. Different procedures are available to do this. The most easily understood approach to solve this problem is the following: N^2 unknown values, the $N \times N$ pixel values of the matrix, have to be computed by solving N_x independent equations, the measured projections. If N_x, the product of the number of projections N_P times the number of data points per projection N_D, is larger than or equal to N^2 this is possible.

In the simplest case of an image matrix with only four pixels (2×2 matrix) two measurements for two projections will yield a system of four equations and four unknowns which can be solved easily (figure 1.6). The extension to a 3×3 matrix with nine unknowns can also be solved easily with twelve measured values given as assumed in this schematic representation. These so-called algebraic reconstruction techniques (ART) were actually used in the early days of CT, as for example in computing the image in figure 1.2a as a 80×80 matrix. The image was computed in an iterative fashion, i.e. by repeating the calculation in an effort to improve accuracy with each step. For larger data volumes, finer image matrices and the higher demand on image quality ART approaches led to unacceptably high computation times.

In today's CT scanners the so-called convolution-backprojection procedure is usually utilized. This is illustrated in figure 1.7. The respective considerations are illustrated additionally by video clips on the CD-ROM which demonstrate the process of image formation in CT. The starting point is always an empty image matrix, i.e. a defined range of computer memory which contains only zeros as starting values. For simple backprojection each projection value is added to all the picture elements in the computer memory along the direction in which it has been measured. (It is possible to reconstruct only a part of the object as a zoom reconstruction. This may improve spatial resolution, as will be discussed in section 4.1.3.) In general, each detail in the object and represented in the attenuation profile does not only contribute to the pixel value at the desired image point, but to the entire image as well. Even when considering only three projections it becomes

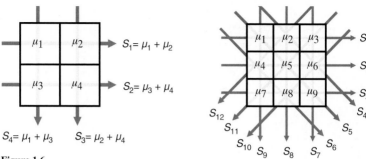

Figure 1.6
How do we compute a CT image?
Algebraic procedures are the most easily comprehensible approach to image reconstruction. The N^2 unknown values of an $N \times N$ image matrix can be determined by solving a system of linear equations. For larger matrices this has to be done iteratively.

apparent that an unsharp image will result. For the very simple object in figure 1.7, the origin of the single image detail is easily recognized, since the image intensity is highest here. The display is unsatisfactory, however, as can be seen in figure 1.7 at the lower left, which represents the result for the chosen object in an actual measurement and reconstruction. The far-reaching signal contributions due to the backprojection process lead to an unsharp image, which is insufficient for the diagnosis of complex structures.

To avoid this unsharpening each projection has to be convoluted before backprojection with a mathematical function, the convolution kernel. This constitutes a pointwise multiplication of the convolution kernel and the attenuation profile and addition of the resulting values (for mathematical definitions see chapter 9.2). In essence, this represents a high pass filtering procedure which generates over- and undershoots at object boundaries. For a positive signal, negative undershoots are generated. These negative contributions will even out the far-reaching positive signal contributions outside each object detail due to the backprojection procedure (figure 1.7 lower right). Convolution additionally offers the possibility to influence image characteristics by the choice and design of the convolution kernel – from soft or smoothing to sharp or edge enhancing (figure 1.8). A relatively weak highpass filter reduces spatial resolution as well as image noise, a strong high pass filter has the opposite effect, as will be discussed further in chapter 4.

Fourier methods offer a further procedure for image reconstruction which is mathematically equivalent to the convolution-backprojection approach. While the ART approach described above is not in practical use anymore in CT, Fourier methods may gain in importance in the future as faster and less costly electronic components become available. Convolution and back-

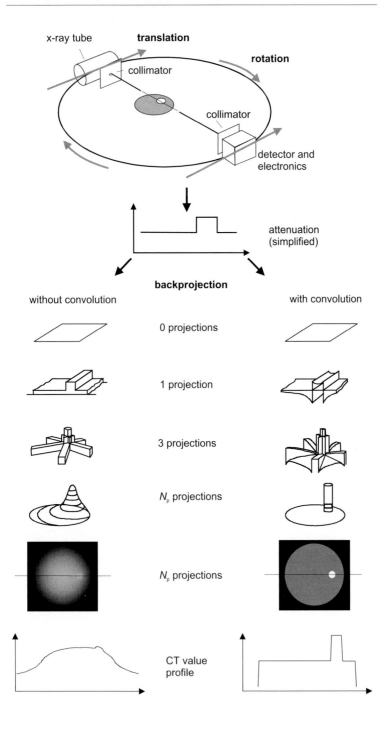

original profile   **convolution kernel**   **filtered profile**

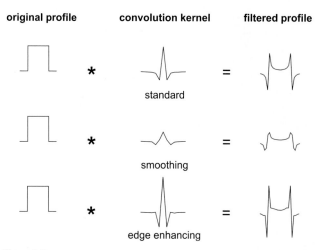

standard

smoothing

edge enhancing

Figure 1.8
Image characteristics can be influenced by the choice of the convolution kernel, whereby increasing spatial resolution or edge enhancement also means increasing image noise.

projection can be considered the method of choice for CT image reconstruction today.

1.2.4   What is displayed in CT Images?

As explained above, CT measures and computes the spatial distribution of the linear attenuation coefficient $\mu(x,y)$. However, the physical quantity μ is not very descriptive and is strongly dependent on the spectral energy used. A display of μ would make quantitative statements cumbersome; a direct comparison of images obtained on scanners with different voltages and filtration would be limited. Therefore, the computed attenuation coefficient is displayed as a so-called CT value relative to the attenuation of water (figure 1.9). In honor of the inventor of CT, CT values, often also referred to as CT numbers, are specified in Hounsfield units (HU). For an arbitrary tissue T with attenuation coefficient μ_T the CT value is defined as

$$\text{CT value} = (\mu_T - \mu_{\text{water}}) / \mu_{\text{water}} \times 1000 \text{ HU} . \tag{1.1}$$

◄ **Figure 1.7**
Image reconstruction in CT by convolution and backprojection.
Direct backprojection of attenuation profiles results in unsharp images. Convolution of attenuation profiles before backprojection, essentially a high pass filtering, counteracts this unsharpening. (See also the video clips on the CD-ROM.)

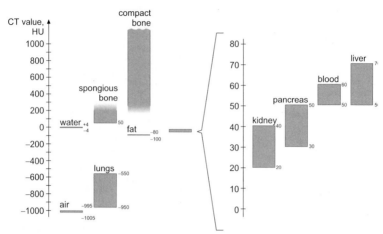

Figure 1.9
The Hounsfield scale. CT values characterize the linear attenuation coefficient of the tissue in each volume element relative to the μ-value of water. The CT values of different tissues are therefore defined to be relatively stable and to a high degree independent of the x-ray spectrum.

On this scale, water and consequently each water-equivalent tissue with $\mu_T = \mu_{water}$, has the value 0 HU by definition. Air corresponds to a CT value of -1000 HU, since $\mu_T = \mu_{air}$ is equal to zero to a good approximation. The CT values of water and air are independent of the energy of the x-rays and therefore constitute the fixed points for the CT value scale.

Lung tissue and fat exhibit negative CT values due to their lower density and the resulting lower attenuation ($\mu_{lung} < \mu_{water}$). Most other body areas exhibit positive CT values, due to the physical density of muscle, connective tissues and most soft tissue organs. For bone and calcifications the higher effective atomic number of calcium, in addition to increased density, is responsible for increased attenuation and therefore for higher CT values of typically up to 2000 HU. CT values of bone or contrast media are more strongly dependent on x-ray energy than water and increase with reduced high voltage settings, which conforms to the contrast behavior in conventional radiographs in principle.

The Hounsfield scale has no upper limit. For medical scanners a range from -1024 HU to $+3071$ HU is typically provided. Consequently, 4096 ($= 2^{12}$) different values are available and 12 bits per pixel are required. Image reconstruction with an extended scale, which is of particular interest for industrial applications, can also be of value in special medical applications. Imaging bone and measuring its density and structure in the vicinity of metallic endoprostheses constitutes one example.

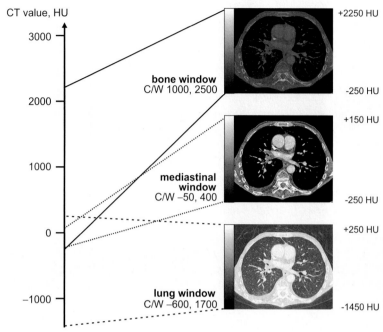

Figure 1.10
Windowing procedures to display CT images. The diagnostically relevant range of CT values is selected by choosing the center and width (C/W) of the window. The complete gray value scale is assigned to this selected range only for display on a monitor or film.

1.2.4.1   Windowing

The CT value range from −1024 HU to +3071 HU, i.e. 4096 gray levels, cannot be evaluated or differentiated in a single view, neither on a monitor nor by documentation on film. Human observers can typically discern up to a maximum of 60 to 80 gray levels. Therefore, the complete gray scale is assigned to the CT value interval of interest only, the so-called window; values above the chosen window will be displayed as white, and the values below the window as black. This procedure, the so-called windowing, is carried out on the CT console interactively and without time delay. To choose the desired CT value interval only the center and the width of the window have to be adjusted by mouse, potentiometer or a similar device. The center is chosen corresponding approximately to the mean CT value of the interesting structures, while the window width determines the contrast in the image. For the display of very small attenuation differences as given in the brain, for example, a narrow window is chosen. For large differences, as presented by the lung or the skeleton, for example, a wide window is chosen (figure 1.10). Examples have been compiled for illustration on the CD-ROM for readers who have no access to a CT scanner or to an evaluation station; these readers can interactively explore the effects of changing window settings using the software package offered there.

1.2.4.2   Significance of CT numbers

CT values can be interpreted in a simple and in most cases unambiguous way. An increase in CT values can be assigned to increased density and/or an increase in effective atomic number. This corresponds to the physical definition of the linear attenuation coefficient

$$\mu = \left(\frac{\mu}{\rho}\right)(E, Z) \cdot \rho \tag{1.2}$$

μ is the product of the density ρ and the mass attenuation coefficient μ/ρ which depends on the energy E of the x-rays used and the atomic number Z of the material or tissue in question. Values of the mass attenuation coefficient as a function of energy are shown in figure 1.11 for several elements and materials relative to the values for water. This illustrates that CT value differences due to effective atomic numbers decrease for higher energies.

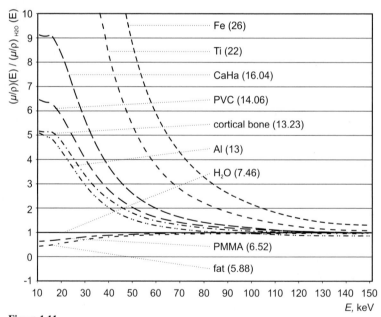

Figure 1.11
Mass attenuation coefficients of different materials relative to those of water; effective atomic numbers are given in parentheses. CT values are increased when the atomic number or the density of the material are higher than that of water.

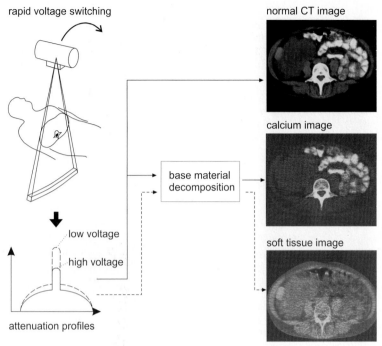

rapid voltage switching

normal CT image

base material
decomposition

low voltage

high voltage

calcium image

soft tissue image

attenuation profiles

Figure 1.12
Principle and results of dual energy CT. The area of increased CT values in the standard
CT image can be interpreted correctly by means of material density images: soft tissue
density is increased, there is no calcium deposit [Kalender, 1987c].

Contrast at high energies is dominated by density differences. This holds
true for tissues of high atomic number, such as bone, in the same way as
for tissues with low atomic numbers, such as fat. The negative contrast of
fat, typically −80 to −100 HU, is caused both by the low effective atomic
number Z_{eff} of approximately 5.88 and by the low density of approximately
0.96 g/cm^3.

For the interpretation of CT values it must also be considered that the contribution of all materials or chemical elements in a given voxel are averaged. The explanation of why attenuation and thus CT values increase or
decrease is nevertheless not a problem in most cases and apparent for
experienced radiologists.

However, there may also be unclear findings, for example the question if a
region with increased attenuation in soft tissue represents a fresh process
corresponding to bleeding or an old process which is diffusely calcified. In
such cases, dual energy CT can clarify the situation (figure 1.12).

Dual energy CT makes use of the energy dependence in μ due to the materials' atomic numbers. In general, two scans with different spectra are carried out and the attenuation values and the differences in attenuation for the two spectra have to be evaluated. Different approaches are available for this purpose. The aim is always to generate material-selective images and to determine material density as accurately as possible. Implementations which are based on the measured attenuation integrals and the principle of base material decomposition can provide images of calcium and soft tissue density (figure 1.12) as well as images of electron density, effective atomic number and so-called monoenergetic images free of beam hardening effects [Kalender, 1987a]. A dual energy CT option was offered for several years on scanners of the SOMATOM DR type and was used especially for the highly accurate measurement of bone mineral density in the lumbar spine. The high technical effort and the increased dose for scans with two different kVp values is not considered adequate anymore today. In technical applications, dual energy methods remain in use, as for example in non-destructive material testing or airport security baggage checks. They will also be considered further for special medical applications, such as the calculation of electron density maps for the planning of radiation therapy.

2 Technical Concepts

2.1 Phases of Development and Goals

The technical goals of CT development have continuously been adapted to the technical state of the art and to the topical demands of radiology. One basic demand has always been of high priority: scan times have to be reduced! In addition to other demands such as improvement of image quality, reduction of costs, adaptation of the user interface etc., which always had to be taken into account also, the reduction of scan times appears to have been the decisive trend pursued since the beginning of CT. The performance and the spectrum of applications developed accordingly, driven or accompanied by the necessary improvements in technology. To a good approximation, although not strictly so, the individual phases of development can be assigned to single decades.

2.1.1 The Seventies – from Head to Whole Body Scanning

The development of CT scanners began with Hounsfield's experimental setup, which largely corresponded to the sketch in figure 1.5. This set-up has often been termed the 'first generation' of CT. The first commercial scanners, the so-called 'second generation', differed only little from Hounsfield's scanning system. To speed up scanning detectors were added, which entailed going from a pencil beam to a small fan beam. Both types of scanners functioned according to the translation-rotation principle in which the radiation source and the detector scan the object in a linear translatory motion and repeat this procedure successively after a small rotational increment (figure 2.1 a,b). In this manner, Hounsfield sampled 180 projections in 1° steps with 160 data points each, i.e. a total of 28,800 data per scan. This was fully sufficient to calculate an image with 6,400 pixels, i.e. an 80 × 80 image matrix. Scan times were five minutes; image reconstruction was carried out simultaneously and took the same amount of time. Hounsfield reported an examination time of 35 minutes, in which the dual-row detector acquired 6 × 2 images with 13 mm slice thickness. This constituted a remarkable performance. In the first trials in 1969 test objects, so-called phantoms, were scanned by Hounsfield with an isotope source and required a scan time of nine days per image.

Most commercial translation-rotation scanners offered a field of measurement for head examinations only. The first attempt to scan whole body cross sections by CT was also based on the translation-rotation principle.

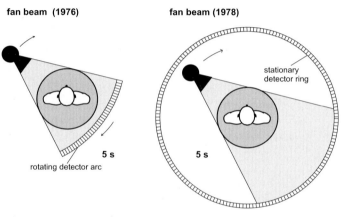

Figure 2.1
From a historical perspective, four scanner generations are known in CT. Head scanners, which scanned the patient by translation and rotation of the measurement system with a pencil beam (**a**) or a small fan beam (**b**), and fan beam systems, in which all body sections can be scanned with a continuous 360° rotation. The '3rd generation', featuring a rotating detector (**c**), has clearly outdistanced the '4th generation', which utilizes stationary detector rings (**d**).

The ACTA scanner (Automatic Computerized Transverse Axial scanner) sampled a field of measurement with 48 cm diameter in a six minute scan. This was sufficient to demonstrate the potential of CT for whole body scanning, but problems due to respiration and patient motion and also to unacceptable total examination times for scanning larger body regions were apparent. In the middle of the seventies the declared goal of technical developments was to reduce the scan time per image to 20 seconds to allow for body scans taken during a single breathhold. The introduction of fan beam scanning was the solution to this problem.

Instead of sampling a transmission profile, i.e. a projection, by a pencil beam with translatory motion, a fan beam and a larger detector arc were used to measure a complete projection simultaneously (figure 2.1c,d). In this approach, the available x-ray power is utilized much more efficiently. The translatory motion becomes obsolete, and the system only executes a rotatory motion. The first whole body scanners with fan beam systems came to the market in 1976, and with these the envisaged goal of 20 seconds per image scan time was achieved. In the first scanners of this type both the x-ray tube and the detector rotated around the patient, demanding higher technical efforts but offering advantages with respect to components cost and image quality ('third generation'). Only a little later scanners followed with a ring-like stationary detector fully encircling the patient, so that only the x-ray tube rotated ('fourth generation'). Rotation systems were quickly accepted, and translation-rotation systems meanwhile disappeared almost completely. The discussion of which type of rotation system is the superior type continues; however, both with respect to numbers installed and, more importantly, with respect to the development of multi-row detectors, which will be discussed below, the third generation has prevailed.

2.1.2   The Eighties – Fast Scanning of Single Slices

For all scanner types it became obvious that image quality and therefore diagnostic capability depended strongly on scan times, since voluntary and involuntary patient motion may lead to losses of image sharpness and to artifacts. The necessary electrical energy was fed to the scanner's x-ray tube by cables. This prevented fast and continuous rotation, since the system had to be accelerated in one direction, stopped after 360° and then accelerated again in the opposite direction. 'Fast scanners' using this technique provided scan times down to two seconds, but in doing so did not altogether fulfill the wishes of radiologists and clinicians.

The goal of providing shorter scan times was pursued in the eighties in the form of many creative approaches. Three different solutions should be mentioned here: conventional systems with the possibility for continuous rotation and data acquisition, electron beam scanners and volume CT scanners. Continuously rotating conventional systems have meanwhile proven to be the most promising approach, while electron beam scanners and other alternative designs have not been able to establish themselves. Section 2.4 discusses the respective developments and other alternative developments.

Continuously rotating CT systems, which were first introduced in 1987 by Siemens Medical Systems (SOMATOM PLUS) and Toshiba Medical Systems (TCT 900S), were based on 'slip ring technology'. The necessary electrical energy for the x-ray tube is transferred by slip rings instead of cables. Consequently, it was possible to abandon the start-stop type of operation (start for clockwise rotation – stop – start for counterclockwise rotation – stop – etc.) and to replace this with continuous data acquisition. This development resulted in decisive new impulses for CT. Not only were scan times reduced to typically one second, but this also provided the basis for advanced dynamic examinations and for spiral CT. The majority of today's CT scanners, of both the 3rd and 4th generation, make use of the principle of continuous rotation.

2.1.3 The Nineties – Fast Volume Scanning

In the year 1990 only one scanner with spiral CT scan mode was available, the Siemens SOMATOM PLUS, which had also been used for the first experimental and clinical trials [Kalender, 1990b]. In 1992, at the annual meeting of the Radiological Society of North America (RSNA) all major CT manufacturers announced scanners with slip ring technology and spiral CT capabilities. Since then an amazing technical development has been observed, providing huge increases in x-ray power, computer capacities and further technical improvements. The modality CT, which had already been considered mature in the eighties, experienced a further 'renaissance', as was widely acknowledged. The introduction of four-slice CT systems with scan times of only 500 ms in the year 1998, which meant a reduction of volume scan times by a factor of 8 compared with the typical 1s system with single-row detector, represents the culmination of these developments for the present. The Elscint Twin, a dual-row detector system introduced in 1994, was a precursor to these developments.

The introduction of multi-row detector systems also seems to mark the end of the 4th CT generation, i.e. scanners with stationary detector rings. The latest and most powerful scanners which are offered commercially today are all 3rd generation scanners, i.e. scanners with rotating detector arrays. We will therefore refer to this type as the "standard scanner configuration" below and explain it in greater detail. Differences and peculiarities of scanners with a stationary detector will be alluded to and discussed wherever required.

Table 2.1 gives a rough overview of the development of some performance characteristics of CT in the course of time, indicating the impressive progress. Only the parameter contrast resolution appears to have reached a plateau very quickly. This is understandable and was to be expected according to physics, since efficient detector systems were available at an early stage. However, it has to be noted that image quality in general and artifact behavior in particular have been improved steadily, which means that since 1980 contrast detectability in clinical images has increased further significantly and steadily.

Table 2.1   Performance characteristics* of CT in a comparison from 1972 to 2000

	1972	1980	1990	2000
Minimum scan time	300 s	5–10 s	1–2 s	0.3–1 s
Data per 360° scan	57.6 kB	1 MB	2 MB	42 MB
Data per spiral scan	–	–	24–48 MB	200–500 MB
Image matrix**	80×80	256×56	512×512	512×512
Power	2 kW	10 kW	40 kW	60 kW
Slice thickness	13 mm	2–10 mm	1–10 mm	0.5–5 mm
Spatial resolution	3 Lp/cm	8–12 Lp/cm	10–15 Lp/cm	12–25 Lp/cm
Contrast resolution	5 mm/5 HU/ 50 mGy	3 mm/3 HU/ 30 mGy	3 mm/3 HU/ 30 mGy	3 mm/3 HU/ 30 mGy

*   Typical values for high performance scanners
** Values refer to the calculated matrix. Monitor displays often use 1024×1024
matrices by means of interpolation.

2.2   Standard Scanner Configuration

2.2.1   Mechanical Design

The two largest single components of a CT unit are the actual examination unit, the so-called gantry, and the patient bed (figure 2.2). They are similar in design for most CT units and determine the minimum floor space required. Further essential components, such as cabinets for electronics, computers and controls, air conditioning etc., are specific to each manufacturer and CT unit and can be placed either in the CT examination room, in a separate service room or in the operator's area. A typical unit is shown in figure 2.2, taking the installation at the Institute of Medical Physics, Erlangen, as an example. Although this represents a scanner of the highest performance class, the SOMATOM Volume Zoom, the space requirements of about 30 m² remain modest.

The actual measuring system, which is hidden in the gantry, is shown schematically in figure 2.3a; the geometry and dimensions given here refer to the specific scanner shown in figure 2.2, but can be taken as typical values. A field of measurement (FOM) of about 50 cm and a gantry opening of about 70 cm, which allow the examination of patients with larger cross-sections, can also be considered as an 'industry standard' in the medium

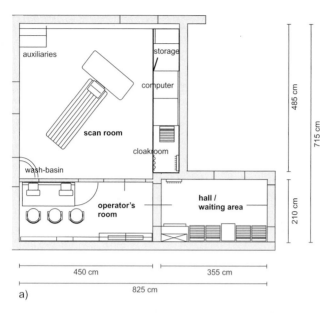

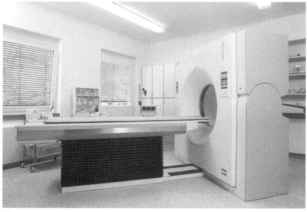

Figure 2.2
Typical CT examination suite (SOMATOM Volume Zoom in the IMP, University of Erlangen).
a) Sketch of the examination room and the operator's area.
b) Photo of the examination room. The patient bed and the gantry, which typically can be tilted by $\pm30°$ and contains the x-ray components and the measuring system, determine the space requirement of about 30 m².

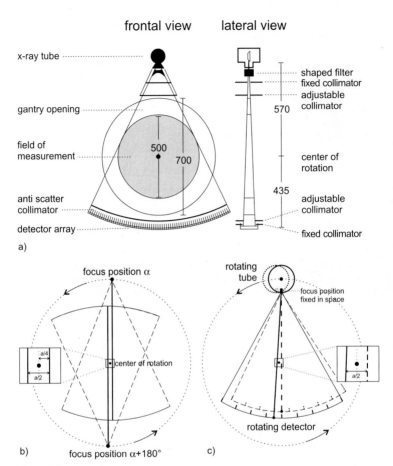

Figure 2.3
Schematic representation of the scanning geometry and important components of the CT measuring system in frontal view (x/y plane) and in lateral view (y/z plane) **(a)**. By misaligning the measuring system by one fourth of the sampling distance, a doubling of the sampling frequency is achieved for 360° measurements **(b)**. An additional similar effect can be reached by use of the so-called flying focus **(c)**.

and upper price segments. The different components and the definition of the fan beam are described in detail below.

The mechanical design of a CT scanner, which may appear to have been a trivial matter for the first CT units, has always imposed high demands on engineering due to the required mechanical accuracy of the sampling process. Among these are the demand for a quarter detector offset to improve sampling, where the distance between the central ray and its direct neighbor measured at the center of rotation is taken as the sampling distance. If the central ray is offset by one fourth of the sampling distance from the center of rotation, then this ray will again be shifted by one fourth of the sampling distance in the opposite direction after 180° rotation. This means that the two measurements with the central ray taken in opposite direction (and in an analogous fashion for all other rays) are offset relative to each other by half the sampling distance (figure 2.3b). The sampling frequency is increased by a factor of two compared with a measurement over 180°. The so-called flying or dynamic focal spot serves a similar purpose. This technical performance feature of some CT x-ray tubes allows controlling the focus position electromagnetically. That is, if the focus is moved on the anode opposite the direction of movement of the x-ray tube, it is then kept fixed in space for two successive measurements. Thereafter the focus 'flies' back to its starting position on the anode, and the process repeats itself. For each focus position in space two measured interlaced projections result, since the detector continues to move continuously. The sampling frequency is thereby doubled (figure 2.3c), thus enhancing the spatial resolution (see section 4.1.3).

The demands on mechanical design have risen continuously with the rotation speeds offered today. The resulting centrifugal forces pose further technological challenges. To appreciate this, one has to take into account that the rotating part of the gantry, i.e. the components shown in figure 2.3a, represent a mass of typically 400–1000 kg. To accelerate these masses to two rotations per second, linear drives integrated into the rotary bearing are preferably used which also guarantee sufficiently uniform motion.

The centrifugal forces which have to expected can be calculated easily. For an x-ray tube to axis of rotation distance of typically 600 mm and a rotation time of 0.5 s per 360° an acceleration of $9.66 \cdot g$ results, i.e. approximately ten times the acceleration due to the earth's gravitational field. For a typical mass of 100 kg of the x-ray tube plus its support, centrifugal forces of nearly 10,000 N have to be balanced out at this point alone. While it is generally known and accepted that other components, such as the x-ray system, detector and image reconstruction system, pose very high demands on technology, this is also the case for mechanical design.

The transfer of electrical energy to the x-ray tube and to the other components on the rotating part of the gantry and data transfer back to the stationary part is mostly achieved by slip rings (figure 2.4). The data from the data acquisition system can alternatively be transferred optically or by high frequency transmission systems. The choice of the respective components will be made according to cost and reliability.

Further functions which the CT system must offer can easily be provided with today's technical means. Among these are the capability of gantry tilt; most CT scanners allow a tilt of the scan plane up to ±30° with respect to the axis of rotation. This allows the selection of scan planes directly

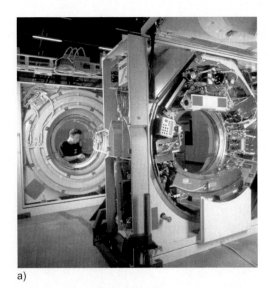

a)

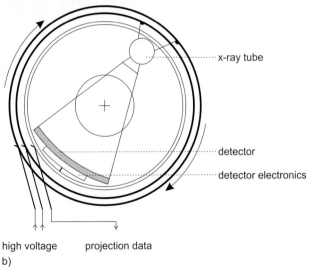

x-ray tube

detector

detector electronics

high voltage   projection data
b)

Figure 2.4
Modern CT systems employ slip ring technology to allow for continuous data acquisition.
a) Photograph of a measuring system during assembly with slip rings (left) and components (right) visible.
b) Schematic representation of slip rings, which allow the transfer of electrical energy to
the x-ray components and data from the detector system to the image reconstruction unit.

through the structures of interest (section 2.3.1), which is important for critical regions, such as the base of the skull or the lumbar spine.

The patient bed essentially has to fulfill two demands: it should allow lowering as far down as possible so that patients can sit on it without any problems, be positioned and then lifted to the actual examination position. The second demand refers to high precision, both for positioning and for table speed. The latter is important for survey radiographs and spiral CT.

2.2.2   X-ray Components

CT has always demanded relatively high x-ray power. This demand has risen dramatically with the increase in scan speed and the introduction of spiral CT. Typical values for the maximum power are 20–60 kW, with the high voltage ranging from 80–140 kVp. The maximum ratings provided by a given system constitute a limit which cannot be sustained over a longer period of time, such as the typical scan times of 30–60 s for spiral CT. In particular the heat storage capacity of anode discs available today would be exceeded, but also the generator capacities, which are mostly adapted in their specifications to the respective x-ray tube. Longer pauses for tube cooling were therefore required for examining larger volumes by sequential single slice scanning. In much the same way, in spiral CT the tube current and thus the power have to be reduced, which often leads to the choice of slice widths thicker than what can be considered optimal. A typical sketch of power versus time is shown in figure 2.5. This documents the dependence of the maximal selectable tube current on the desired spiral scan duration.

These technical limitations, which will remain for the foreseeable future, explain the particular attractiveness of multi-row detector systems. The available x-ray power is used much more efficiently, since M slices offer a solid angle which is M times larger than for a single one. To a first approximation, the scan duration will be reduced by this factor M and allow for a selection of higher power settings. Alternatively, multi-row detectors may allow the utilization of x-ray components with correspondingly reduced power ratings at lower cost. This does not appear generally desirable, since high power ratings are obligatory for many special applications and for single slice scans as will be seen.

X-ray tubes used in CT today offer focal spot sizes of typically 0.5 to 2.0 mm. Often, a selection of foci is available. The SOMATOM Volume Zoom, for example, offers two focus sizes of 0.8 mm × 1.2 mm and 0.7 mm × 0.9 mm. Smaller foci are preferable for scans with thin slices and high resolution; for scans of large volumes with the primary aim of high soft tissue or contrast resolution, larger focus size with higher power ratings are desirable (figure 2.5). The optional performance feature of a 'flying' focus, which allows controlling the focus position on the anode during the scan, has already been alluded to in the previous section.

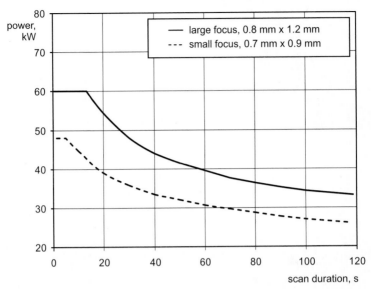

Figure 2.5
Maximal x-ray power depends on scan duration and prior tube load. For spiral scans of long duration power has to be reduced to avoid excessive loading. The reduction of total scan time offered by multi-row detectors allows reduction of tube loading or, alternatively, the selection of higher power values and/or the choice of the thin slice settings necessary for high 3D-resolution.

2.2.3 Collimators and Filtration

CT systems feature various collimators, filters and shielding designs which provide filtration of the x-ray spectra, definition of the measured slices, guarding the detector against scattered radiation and general radiation protection (figure 2.3a). They may vary from scanner type to scanner type, but in principle they always offer the same functions. A first collimation is provided very close to the focus to reduce the generated radiation roughly to the maximally anticipated beam for the given detector and geometry. This first reduction of the radiation cone is provided by the lead housing of the x-ray tube itself, which provides an aperture for rough definition of the fan beam. In a second step the maximum permitted fan is defined exactly by a fixed collimator. An additional adjustable collimator allows variable collimation to the desired slice width. The latter collimator is placed as far from the focus as possible, i.e. close to the gantry housing, to minimize penumbral regions caused by the finite focus size.

The influence of collimator geometry and focus size on the definition of the slice is illustrated in figure 2.6. For an ideal point focus a perfect rectangular slice profile results. For any real extended focus penumbral regions and, to a first approximation, a trapezoidal profile result. The

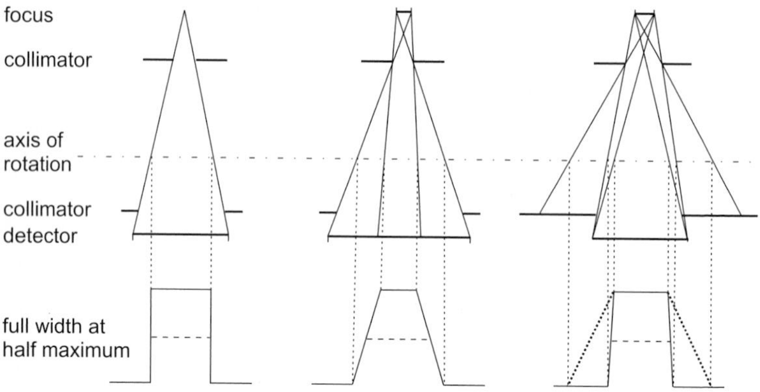

Figure 2.6
Definition of the scanned slice. The width and profile of the exposed slice are determined by the focus size, collimator geometry and width. The use of a detector collimator (right) will have a positive influence on the slice profile (solid), whereas the dose profile (dotted) will remain wide and therefore exceed the slice profile.

deviation from a rectangle can be reduced by a movable collimator in front of the detector; such means are used in particular for defining very thin slices, since here the highest relative deviations from the ideal rectangular form have to be expected. It must be accepted, however, that the dose profile will be wider than the sensitivity profile. This simply reflects the situation that the exposed section is thicker than the section measured by the detector (figure 2.6 right). The considerations for measuring and assessing slice sensitivity profiles and dose profiles and aspects of multi-slice scanning will be discussed further in chapters 4 and 5.

Collimators in front of the detector – in addition to the optional movable collimator there is always a fixed collimator with a width corresponding to the maximum collimation – serve to minimize signal contributions from scattered radiation. Optional antiscatter collimators serve the same function, reducing contributions from scattered radiation; these are mostly implemented as a system of thin lamellae made of strongly absorbing material, e.g. 100 μm thick tantalum sheets, which are positioned between the single detector elements and aligned exactly in the direction of the x-ray focus. This alignment, although technically demanding, is necessary to avoid a reduction of signal-carrying primary radiation and can only be implemented in scanners with a rotating detector. Scanners with stationary detector rings (4th generation) in consequence suffer a severe disadvantage with respect to the suppression of scattered radiation. This can be considered as one reason why, apart from a dual-row detector system for electron beam CT (see section 2.4.1), multi-row detector systems are not offered with stationary detectors.

Several components add to the filtration of the x-ray spectrum. In addition to the inherent filtration of the x-ray tube, which typically amounts to 3 mm aluminum-equivalent thickness, flat or shaped filters are also used. Flat filters, for example copper sheets of 0.1 to 0.4 mm thickness, shift the spectrum to higher energies. Low energy portions, which contribute strongly to the dose, but less to the signal, are reduced to a high degree. The use of additional filtration is therefore welcomed, but also demands higher x-ray power.

So-called shaped or 'bow-tie' filters attenuate radiation hardly at all in the center, but strongly in the periphery (figure 2.3a frontal view). They reduce the demands on the dynamic range of the detector system and scattered radiation intensities arising from peripheral object zones, and also the patient dose. The material for shaped filters should be of low atomic number in order to keep the spectral and beam hardening differences between the center and the periphery of the fan beam as small as possible. Teflon, for example, is an efficient filter material for this purpose due to its high density combined with a relatively low effective atomic number.

One further component of the collimator system, which is employed close to the detector in some systems, is the so-called 'high-resolution comb'. The teeth of the comb overlap with the gaps between detector elements and, depending on their width, reduce the detector aperture W_D to improve spatial resolution (see section 4.1.3). It is clear that this will also reduce the geometric dose efficiency of the total system. Such devices are therefore only used for high contrast scanning, where increased noise does not pose a particular problem.

2.2.4   Detector Systems

The detector, the system for quantitative recording of the incident ionizing radiation, constitutes one of the most important and technologically most critical components of the entire CT system. It has to transform the incident x-ray intensity into a corresponding electrical signal, to amplify this signal and to convert it from analog to digital form. The decisive components are the x-ray sensitive detector elements and their geometrical configuration, the preamplifiers and the analog-to-digital converters. The demands on the electronics, i.e. preamplifiers and analog-to-digital converters (ADC), can be specified relatively easily. The electronic noise level generated by these components should be significantly lower than the statistical fluctuations in x-ray intensities due to quantum noise. A frequently stated requirement is that the electronic noise must not be higher than half the magnitude of the maximally expected quantum noise, i.e. $\sigma_E < 0.5\sigma_Q$. Several other characteristics of the detector system and their evaluation are more difficult to specify, however. Some of the essential demands are summarized in table 2.2.

Table 2.2 Demands on CT detector systems

Demands on CT detector systems	Acceptable values
High dynamic range	10^5–10^6
High linearity over the complete dynamic range	
High quantum absorption efficiency	> 90 % (ideally 100 %)
High luminescence efficiency* for scintillation detectors	> 5 % (ideally 100 %)
High geometric efficiency	80 %–90 % (ideally 100 %)
Fast temporal response and decay	Decay constant < 10 μs
Low afterglow	< 0.01 %, 100 ms after end of irradiation
Low radiation drift	$\leq$ 0.5 % for longest scan duration
Electronic noise low compared with quantum noise for all scan modes	$\sigma_E \leq 0.5 \cdot \sigma_Q$
Low crosstalk between detector elements	< 3 %
High homogeneity of the material of each detector element for good artifact behavior	i.e. purity of the material > 99.99 %
Equal response of all detector elements within a detector array	< 0.1 % difference (after optional correction)
Detector material machinable in a simple manner with high precision	± 10 μm tolerance
Feasibility for configuration as single or multi-row array	$D \geq 4$ rows
Environmental acceptability of the detector material	Low toxicity, low disposal cost
Chemical stability	e.g. resistant to moisture
Stable against environmental influences	e.g. thermal expansion coefficient < 10^{-5} per °C
Feasibility of collimation against scattered radiation	
Low cost and easy to service	

*   Ratio of the energy of visible light to be detected
   to the energy of the absorbed x-ray intensity

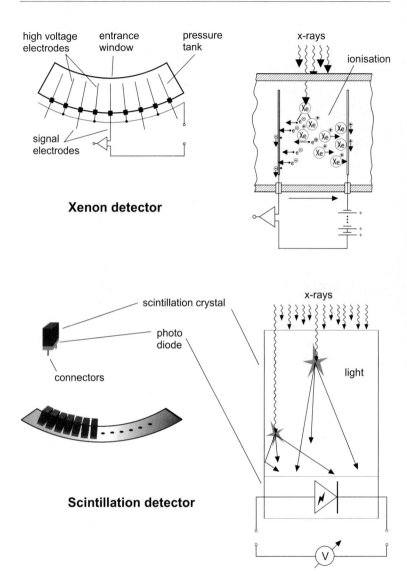

Figure 2.7
Two detector systems dominate CT:
a) xenon ionization chambers,
b) scintillation detectors.

For the implementation of detectors, many approaches have been discussed and pursued. In CT two conversion principles and detector types have predominantly been set to use:

- Ionization chambers, mostly filled with the noble gas xenon under high pressure

- Scintillation detectors in the form of crystals, such as cesium iodide or cadmium tungstate, and ceramic materials, such as gadolinium oxysulfide.

A sketch of these two detector types and their operating principles is shown in figure 2.7. Semiconductor materials, solid state detectors which provide an electrical signal directly and are therefore often called direct converters, have not been used in clinical scanners until now. Such developments are not expected in the short term.

Xenon ionization chambers (figure 2.7a) offer several advantages: their construction is relatively simple in principle, and the sensitivity of the individual detector channels is exactly the same since constant gas pressure exists for the complete detector pressure chamber. The temporal response of xenon, with fast decay and low afterglow, has frequently been cited as a further decisive advantage. Temporal characteristics will be explained and discussed below in comparison to solid state systems.

Lower quantum efficiency has to be listed as a disadvantage of xenon detectors in comparison with solid state detector materials. This does not mean in general, however, that xenon systems are necessarily inferior to scintillator systems. All factors of influence must be taken into account. The total efficiency of the detector system is not given by the quantum absorption efficiency of the detector material and depth alone, since a number of additional factors also contribute. Geometric efficiency is also essential and mostly determined by the dead spaces between the individual elements. These are typically of the order of 0.1 to 0.2 mm in the fan direction for detector element widths of 1 to 2 mm. Xenon detectors may vary strongly in their performance depending on the design: their efficiency may vary drastically, depending on the pressure, chamber depth, thickness of the entrance window and other construction details (table 2.3).

Image quality in general, in particular detector-dependent artifact behavior, influences low-contrast detectability and thus also directly or indirectly the dose efficiency of the complete system. Xenon detectors offer advantages in this respect due to their homogeneous gas distribution and the resultant uniform response. This explains why they were considered the system of choice for a long time. In combination with their temporal response, this also explains why some manufacturers changed their systems from solid state detectors to xenon in the late eighties when faster systems were demanded.

Table 2.3 Detector efficiency for typical detector systems

Object Detector	20 cm H_2O	20 cm H_2O and 2 cm bone	40 cm H_2O and 4 cm bone
120 kVp			
Xenon[1] (10 bar, 3 cm)	42.8 %	39.2 %	32.9 %
Xenon[1] (25 bar, 6 cm)	73.8 %	74.0 %	72.7 %
Ceramic scintillator[2]	89.9 %	88.1 %	84.5 %
140 kVp			
Xenon[1] (10 bar, 3 cm)	38.4 %	34.3 %	27.1 %
Xenon[1] (25 bar, 6 cm)	71.0 %	70.3 %	67.0 %
Ceramic scintillator[2]	85.3 %	83.0 %	78.2 %

[1] 1.3 mm aluminum entrance window, chamber pressure and depth given in parentheses
[2] Gadolinium oxysulfide with 1.4 mm depth

The demand for very short decay times has gained in importance with the introduction of subsecond scan times. To illustrate this point, figure 2.8a shows decay curves for some typical detector materials. The temporal decay of a signal after a short radiation pulse is determined in essence by two phenomena: a. by its decay, the rapid exponential falloff of the largest signal components, and b. by its afterglow, a second much slower decay phase with smaller signal contributions which can also be approximated by a multiexponential function. The superior characteristics of UFC (Ultra Fast Ceramic), a sintered ceramic gadolinium oxysulfide (Gd_2O_2S) material with a decay time of 10^{-6} s, are evident. Their effect on spatial resolution and image quality can be demonstrated by means of simulation. For this purpose measured data of a SOMATOM PLUS 4 with UFC detector were manipulated in the following way: to each of the measured data obtained in intervals of 0.5 ms, an afterglow contribution was added according to the function $\exp(-t/\tau)$. Even for a decay constant $\tau = 1$ ms a significant smoothing influence on anatomic structures becomes visible (figure 2.8b).

This influence of the decay characteristics on spatial resolution has also been verified in a direct comparison of a UFC detector and a xenon detector in an otherwise unchanged CT system; a significant improvement in

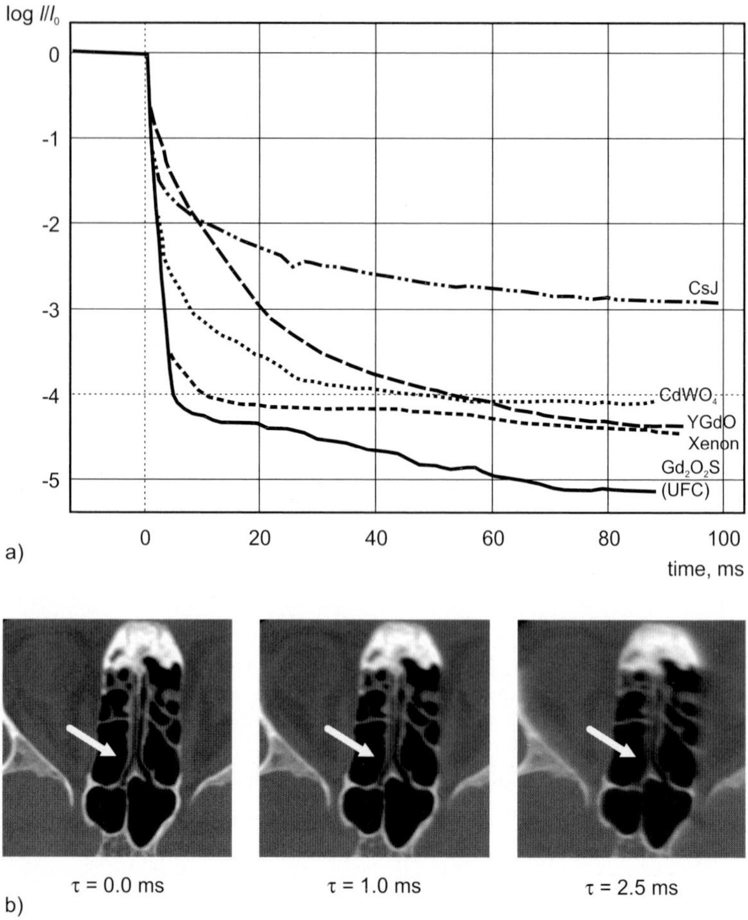

a)

τ = 0.0 ms   τ = 1.0 ms   τ = 2.5 ms

b)

Figure 2.8
Temporal response of detectors.
a) Decay characteristics of different detector materials after a short x-ray pulse.
b) Slow signal decay may influence image quality, in particular spatial resolution, in a
negative way. Simulations of this effect demonstrate that this is already the case for a
decay constant τ = 1 ms.

spatial resolution was found to result for the UFC detector [Fuchs, 1999].
Any advantage with respect to image quality amounts directly to an advantage with respect to dose efficiency, as will be discussed further in chapter
5; accordingly, temporal response has to be considered an important detector characteristic with respect to dose in addition to quantum efficiency. In

Table 2.4 CT scanners with multi-row detector systems. D represents the number of detector rows, M the number of simultaneously scanned slices.

Manufacturer	Scanner type	No. of rows D	No. of slices M	Year
EMI	Mark I	2	2	1972
Siemens	SIRETOM 2000	2	2	1974
Siemens	SOMATOM SD	2	2	1977
Imatron	C-100	2	2	1983
Elscint	Twin	2	2	1994
GE	LightSpeed	16	4	1998
Siemens	SOMATOM Volume Zoom	8	4	1998
Marconi	Mx8000	8	4	1998
Toshiba	Aquilion	34	4	1998

any case, for the high scan speeds reached today, xenon detectors are no longer considered to be the gold standard of today's technology.

A further disadvantage of xenon detectors – and this may possibly be the decisive disadvantage with respect to future developments – is the fact that linear arrays for single-slice scanning can be built very easily, but multi-row designs or complete arrays are extremely difficult to manufacture. Accordingly, all multi-row detectors in the past and all new detector systems have been built with ceramics or scintillation crystals (table 2.4).

High geometric efficiency is a requirement for detectors which has particular importance for multi-row detectors. This implies that dead spaces should be as small as possible. The septa and, whenever in use, the anti-scatter collimators between the individual detector elements which are oriented towards the focus, have a width of typically 0.1 to 0.2 mm, while the separation of elements in the z-direction is approximately 0.1 mm. Values of geometric efficiency of 80 to 90 % are therefore the best available today. For arrays with a finer separation of detector elements in the z-direction a stronger reduction of geometric efficiency must be accepted.

Examples for multi-row detector arrays are shown in figure 2.9. Due to cost considerations complete separate electronic channels are not provided for each individual detector element. Whenever slice thicknesses larger than the minimum thickness given by the array pitch are selected, the signal from several elements is combined in the z-direction, amplified and A/D-converted. This implies the capability to define the slice width by an

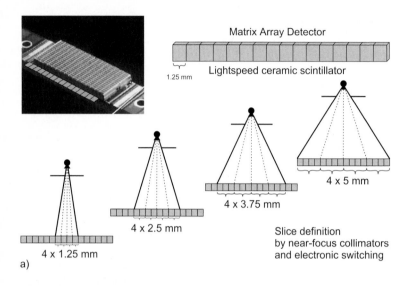

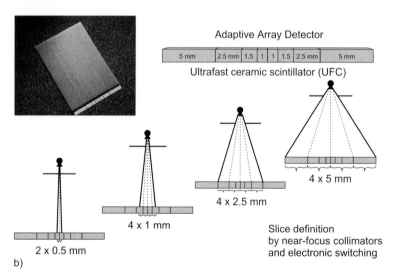

Figure 2.9
Multi-row detector systems for spiral CT.
The number of the slices scanned simultaneously and their width are defined by pre-patient collimation and post-patient electronic combination of signals from the detector array.
a) Isotropically structured detector array (GE LightSpeed).
b) Anisotropically structured detector array (Siemens SOMATOM Volume Zoom and Marconi Mx8000).

electronic combination of signals, whereas the x-ray beam is collimated close to the x-ray source in the usual way.

Figure 2.9a shows the technical solution which GE Medical Systems presently offers. The 16 individual rows of the detector array which offer a minimum slice thickness of 1.25 mm at the center of rotation can be combined to single slices of 1.25 mm, 2.5 mm, 3.75 mm or 5 mm, respectively. Toshiba Medical Systems offers a similar solution of a more or less isotropically structured matrix array in a technically more demanding way with a 34-row array design for its Aquilion. The innermost four rows define a 0.5 mm slice each, followed on each side by 15 rows of 1 mm. Here also, only four slices can be measured simultaneously, i.e. in this case four slices of 0.5 mm, 1 mm, 2 mm, 4 mm or 8 mm, respectively.

An alternative solution which in principle represents a similar approach, but attempts to minimize dead spaces, was developed by Siemens in cooperation with Elscint and is provided in the SOMATOM Volume Zoom and in the Marconi Mx8000. The design of such a so-called adaptive array is shown in figure 2.9b, where only the two innermost detector rows define thin 1 mm slices directly, while offering increasing slice widths off center. Here also, slices are defined by pre-patient collimation and the post-patient combination of measured signals. Of course additional post-patient collimation is always possible also. An important advantage of an adaptive array of this type is that the outermost thicker slices, in this case 5 mm slices, do not contain septa and do not cause a reduction in geometric efficiency. A definition of very thin slices is possible by narrowing the pre-patient collimation and limitation to only the two innermost detector rows.

Both detector concepts presented here, regularly structured isotropic and "adaptive" anisotropic arrays, represent decisive technological advances which will characterize CT in the years ahead. An expansion to higher numbers of rows and slices will require greater efforts and investment with respect to detector electronics. Arrays expanded in the z-direction constitute a continuous transition from fan beam to cone beam. They require further efforts with respect to image reconstruction and data corrections to reduce or eliminate a negative influence on image quality due to the increasing cone beam angles. The contributions from scattered radiation will also increase drastically. These problems are discussed in section 2.4.3.

2.3   Scan Modes and Scan Parameters

The routine operation of a CT scanner requires only a few scan modes. These can be operated with a wide range of parameter settings. A routine examination simply requires taking a survey radiograph for orientation over the anatomy in question, selecting slices or scan regions and scanning them in the sequential or spiral CT mode.

2.3.1   Survey Radiographs

To select the position of single slices or complete scan regions it has proven very helpful to generate a survey radiograph similar to a conventional radiograph. For this purpose the x-ray tube is kept in a fixed angular position and the patient is transported through the field of measurement at low speed, with radiation emitted continuously or in pulsed mode. Digital survey radiographs with high dynamic range, but only low spatial resolution, result. They are mostly taken in a.p. or p.a. direction, or as lateral projections (figure 2.10). In principle, any projection angle can be chosen. Lateral views are of particular interest to select the gantry tilt according to anatomy. For example, slices parallel to the base of the skull or placed exactly in the intervertebral spaces of the lumbar spine can be selected precisely in this way. In most cases the patient is positioned automatically for the slices or scan regions selected in the survey radiograph to be acquired. This helps to speed up the examination, but also serves in the interest of radiation protection since the survey radiograph – often called the topogram, scout view or scanogram – is taken with very low dose. In most cases, they eliminate the need for CT scans which would have to be taken simply for orientation. Survey radiographs can also be used to document the scanned slices and regions.

2.3.2   Scanning Single Slices – Sequential CT

For more than two decades CT examinations consisted of scanning single slices sequentially. In general this meant scans over 360°; partial scans over 180° (for parallel beam geometry with first and second generation scanners) or typically 240° (180° plus fan angle for fan beam geometry) are possible as well. After scanning a single slice, the patient is transported for a defined distance or scan increment, mostly selected equal to the chosen slice thickness. Then the next scan is taken and the procedure is repeated. This examination mode, which meanwhile has been largely replaced by spiral CT, is relatively time-demanding since time is required for table feed and, in many cases, breathing commands. Examination of complete organs will typically take from five to twenty minutes in this way.

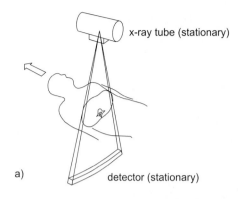

x-ray tube (stationary)

a)

detector (stationary)

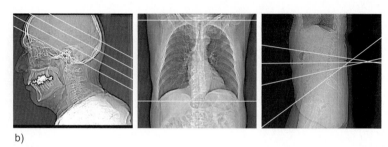

b)

Figure 2.10
Digital survey radiographs are taken with low dose and low spatial resolution by transporting the patient through the field of measurement with the x-ray tube in a fixed position **(a)**. The projection direction (here a.p.) is arbitrary in principle. Survey radiographs allow the selection of the position and gantry tilt for single slices or complete scan regions as shown schematically **(b)**.

Modern scanners offer automated and therefore fast modes for scanning single slices sequentially. In addition to the time necessary for table feed and breathing commands, fundamental disadvantages remain: overlapping images, which are important for high 3D image quality (see section 4.2.4), are generally not available. Nevertheless, indications for single slice scanning will remain. Whenever single scans are required for orientation or whenever representative slices at larger scan increments are indicated, such as in some lung examinations, sequential scanning will continue to be used. Dynamic CT and interventional CT (see below) will also continue to require the capability for single slice scanning.

Sequential partial scan examinations may become more important for cardiac imaging with very fast scanners. A minimum scan range of 180° plus the fan angle is required to measure all line integrals at least once in fan beam geometry [Parker, 1982]. This means, for example, that prospectively triggered scans of the heart can be taken in about 0.3 s on a 0.5 s rotation

Table 2.5 Scan parameters for sequential single-slice CT

Parameter	Symbol	Typical values
Voltage	U	80 to 140 kVp
Tube current	I	10 to 500 mA
Power	P	10 to 60 kW
Slice thickness	S	0.5 to 10 mm
Scan time per 360°	t	0.5 to 2.0 s
Scan increment	SI	Arbitrary, mostly $SI = S$
Number of slices	N_{rot}	10 to 60
Scan range	R	5 to 100 cm $R = (N_{rot} - 1) \cdot SI + S$

scanner, which in most cases yields scans essentially free of motion arti-facts in the diastolic phase. Current work using ECG-based triggering will be discussed in chapter 7.

The parameters generally used for single-slice scanning are summarized in table 2.5. They are valid also to a large degree for all other scan modes described below.

2.3.3   Material-selective Imaging – Dual-Energy CT

Dual-energy methods serve to obtain information about the material com-position in the tissues examined (see section 1.2.4.2). To achieve this a selected slice is scanned with two different spectra, i.e. with different high voltage values and possibly with different filtration. This can be done in two successive scans or by switching the high voltage rapidly from projec-tion to projection. The physically most rigorous approach to data proces-sing consists of the so-called base material decomposition of the measured attenuation data; this allows, for example, calculating images of water- and calcium-equivalent density (figure 1.11) or calculating images representing electron density and effective atomic number [Kalender, 1987a]. This option, which was provided on scanners of the type Siemens SOMATOM DR for a long time, is no longer offered commercially since no significant diagnostic advantages were shown. But there is still some interest, for example, in using electron density images for radiation therapy planning, particularly for proton therapy, with its higher demands on accuracy.

2.3.4   Serial Scanning – Dynamic CT

Dynamic CT is used to record temporal changes in the attenuation characteristics of the object examined. Such changes may represent physiological processes, such as heart motion or breathing. In clinical applications the assessment of contrast medium dynamics in various body regions is of the greatest interest. Typically, a representative slice, or M slices for multi-slice scanners, respectively, are selected, contrast medium is administered and the selected slices are scanned repeatedly. The time interval between single scans depends on the physiological process to be examined and the type of contrast medium. This is illustrated for the example of measurements of brain tissue perfusion in section 7.1, where either the enhancement of xenon is recorded by scans in one-minute intervals during continuous inhalation or the passage of an intravenously injected contrast medium bolus is measured with the highest possible temporal resolution.

In a wider sense, dynamic CT is also realized in cases of multiphase examinations of complete organs after contrast medium injection. Scanning the liver in the early arterial, the portovenous and the late venous phase is a frequently cited example. Such examinations, which have become possible with spiral CT, will become even more practical with multi-slice spiral CT systems. Their higher performance will add to the importance of dynamic CT.

2.3.5   CT Fluoroscopy – Interventional CT

Minimally invasive therapy approaches have continuously gained in importance in recent years; the development of advanced technologies for image-based and image-guided interventions has made a significant contribution to this. Interventions are now frequently carried out in the CT examination room. One prerequisite is the generation of images in approximately real time, corresponding to fluoroscopic methods in conventional radiology.

Monitoring interventions by CT can be carried out with single scans taken at larger time intervals in many cases. The term CT fluoroscopy mostly refers to the continuous scanning of a slice, as with dynamic CT, but with the fastest possible reconstruction and presentation of images. To follow the demand of real-time presentation to as close an approximation as possible, reduced matrices are calculated in many cases, typically 256×256 instead of 512×512. In this way frequencies of five or even more images per second have become possible, allowing the monitoring of many interventions continuously and practically in real time.

2.3.6   Volume Scanning – Spiral CT

Spiral CT means the fast and continuous scanning of complete volumes; it replaces the sequential scanning of single slices, which means only discrete sampling along the z-axis. The technical prerequisites for its implementation have been provided by the introduction of slip ring technology in continuously rotating scanners. The scanning principle (figure 3.2), technical aspects and questions regarding image reconstruction will be discussed in detail in chapter 3. Slip ring technology, the prerequisite for spiral CT, is meanwhile widely used in scanners with rotating detector systems as well as in scanners with stationary detectors and also in so-called compact or low-cost scanners. The differences are seen with respect to performance characteristics. The x-ray power provided, the detector system and the capacity of the computer system all decisively influence the performance of the scanners. Modern systems with multi-row detectors and rotation times in the subsecond range allow the scanning of complete organs or anatomical regions within a few seconds and therefore meet almost all clinical demands with respect to routine applicability and adequate patient comfort.

2.4 Alternative Scanner Concepts

In the following section technical approaches are described and discussed which until now have not been in clinical use at all or only to a limited extent. In part, the solutions are considered exotic due to image quality problems and other disadvantages or they are considered not economical due to increased effort and costs. Nevertheless, to describe and to discuss such concepts in detail is not only of interest for the sake of completeness, but may also enable us to predict future trends in several respects.

2.4.1 Electron Beam CT

Electron beam scanners were already proposed in 1977 with the declared goal to provide extremely short scan times for examinations of the heart. In keeping with this goal, they were initially promoted as cardiovascular CT (CVCT) scanners [Boyd, 1983]. The revolutionary concept was to scan without mechanical motion. For this an electron beam is generated, accelerated, focussed and steered electromagnetically over the anode, a ring-like target enclosing the patient (figure 2.11a). A partial scan over 216° is completed in 50 to 100 milliseconds and can be repeated with practically no delay. The first CT scanner of this design was developed by D.P. Boyd and was introduced to the market by Imatron Inc.; several dozen of these units are in clinical use today. Electron beam tomography (EBT, EBCT), often called cine CT or ultrafast CT (UFCT), aims at covering the complete spectrum of radiological diagnosis. The focus is still on cardiac applications, however.

The general acceptance and broad clinical use of EBT was prevented in the eighties and nineties by the high cost and by the limitations in image qual-

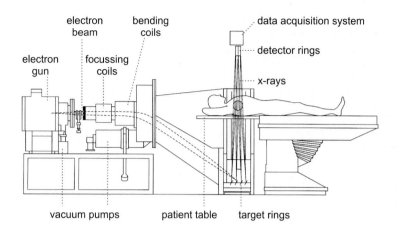

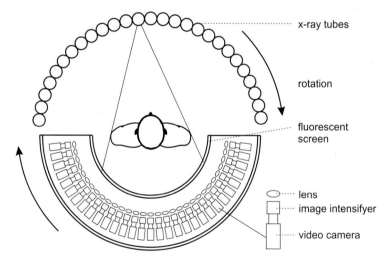

Figure 2.11
Alternative concepts for fast volume scanning.
a) Electron beam tomography permits scans in the range of 50 to 100 ms without mechanical motion.
b) The 'Dynamic Spatial Reconstructor' allowed volume scanning in cone beam geometry with rotation times of only 1 second.

ity. These problems have not been overcome so far, and new developments in this area are not likely since multi-slice spiral CT has meanwhile proven to be superior with respect to image quality and scan speed per volume. Even imaging of the heart, which was considered a domain of EBT due to its short scan time per single slice, is possible in high quality with conventional scanners having subsecond scan times and multi-slice spiral capability (see sections 3.4.3 and 7.3). The idea of scanning without mechanical motion and with arbitrarily short scan times will nevertheless continue to stimulate the imagination of physicists and engineers.

2.4.2   The "Dynamic Spatial Reconstructor"

A completely different approach to fast volume scanning was pursued by R.A. Robb and co-workers [Robb, 1983], who aimed at using conventional technology. In an apparently gigantic setup they planned to have 28 x-ray tubes and 28 fluorescent screens rotate continuously around the patient (figure 2.11b). Instead of scanning single slices successively, they proposed a cone beam geometry to cover a complete volume in only one rotation. The scanner was actually built in a scaled-down version with 'only' 14 x-ray tubes for physiological animal experiments at the Mayo Clinic in Rochester, Minnesota, and allowed the simultaneous acquisition of 240 slices with 0.9 mm slice width. The total scan time of this gigantic setup, weighing many tons, was actually only one second. Officially it was called the Dynamic Spatial Reconstructor in the literature; some critics called it the 'Mayo Monster' due to its physical dimensions.

The technical concept was not pursued further due to cost and effort, technical problems and due to absolutely unsatisfactory image quality compared with standard CT. However, even if not fully intended at that point in time, it defined the goal for future CT developments: the scanning of larger volumes in shorter time with even thinner slices, i.e. with almost isotropic spatial resolution, allowing for dynamic volume scanning at the same time. The essential idea is to use a true area detector for CT data acquisition instead of a single or multi-row detector array.

2.4.3   Cone Beam CT

The transition from scanning one or only a few slices to data acquisition for an entire field means the transition from fan beam to cone beam geometry. The underlying considerations represent a decisive future-oriented development for computed tomography. Various approaches to this goal are under investigation today; nevertheless, a solution which would lend itself to clinical CT imaging with its high demands on image quality and, in particular, low-contrast detectability has not yet been established.

There is no exact definition in the literature for when a fan beam, assumed to be planar, becomes a cone beam. For the clinical systems in use today, for example, strict planar geometry is always assumed, even for four fans although they cover up to 4×8 mm in z-direction. It may therefore be appropriate not to base the definition on the detector or the type of scanning, but instead on the type of reconstruction. For all multi-slice scanners in use today an ideal fan beam geometry is assumed; there are no additional assumptions with respect to geometry or corrections for divergence of the fan. A 2D-reconstruction (see section 9.2.2) is simply applied in all cases. Whenever the non-planar geometry is taken into account and a 3D-reconstruction is carried out (see section 9.2.3) we refer to this as cone beam CT.

The principal problem inherent in cone beam geometry is illustrated in figure 2.12a. Details in the object are projected onto different detector rows for different projection angles, depending on their distance from the central plane. The data recorded in a 360° rotation by an off-center detector row no longer represent a planar slice, as expected for single-row detectors and as is apparently still the case to a sufficiently good approximation for multi-slice scanning up to $M = 4$ corresponding to a maximum cone angle of about 1°. Here opposing rays are still offset by a distance ΔS less than one slice width at the edge of the field of measurement; since the offset decreases further towards the center, $\Delta S > S$ may be considered an acceptable criterion to assure acceptable image quality in multi-slice CT.

The data sets recorded by any single row in cone beam geometry will become increasingly inconsistent with increasing distance of the specific row from the central plane. If this is ignored, artifacts will result whenever the cone angle exceeds a few degrees. For this reason, true cone beam CT with area detectors is employed in practice today only when compromises with respect to image quality are permitted. This is mostly the case for high contrast displays, which require high spatial resolution, but do not require the degree of freedom from artifacts necessary for low-contrast detail detectability. Examples are the imaging of vessels after administering contrast medium, preferably by an intraarterial injection, or applications in non-destructive material testing in medicine or industry. Examples of these are shown in figure 2.12b, c.

In both cases conventional area detectors were used. 3D-CT angiography scans (figure 2.12b) were acquired with a rotating C-arm and standard image intensifier after intraarterial injection [Fahrig, 1997]. This application has meanwhile reached product status (Siemens Multistar with 3D-Angio option). It only allows the assessment of vascular anatomy and pathology, but not of soft tissues, which exhibit low contrast. The micro-CT examination of a bone biopsy (figure 2.12c) was taken with a 1024 × 1024 CCD array [Kalender, 1997; Engelke, 1999]. Today, micro-CT scanners are also commercially available. In both cases an approximate 3D-image reconstruction of the Feldkamp algorithm type (see section 9.2.3) is employed. Spatial resolution is extremely high, consistent with the given task and the implementation using about 100 μm and 10 μm effective detector element dimensions, respectively. The requirements for low-contrast detectability, which would have to be provided by a clinical CT scanner, have not yet been fulfilled. New reconstruction procedures (see section

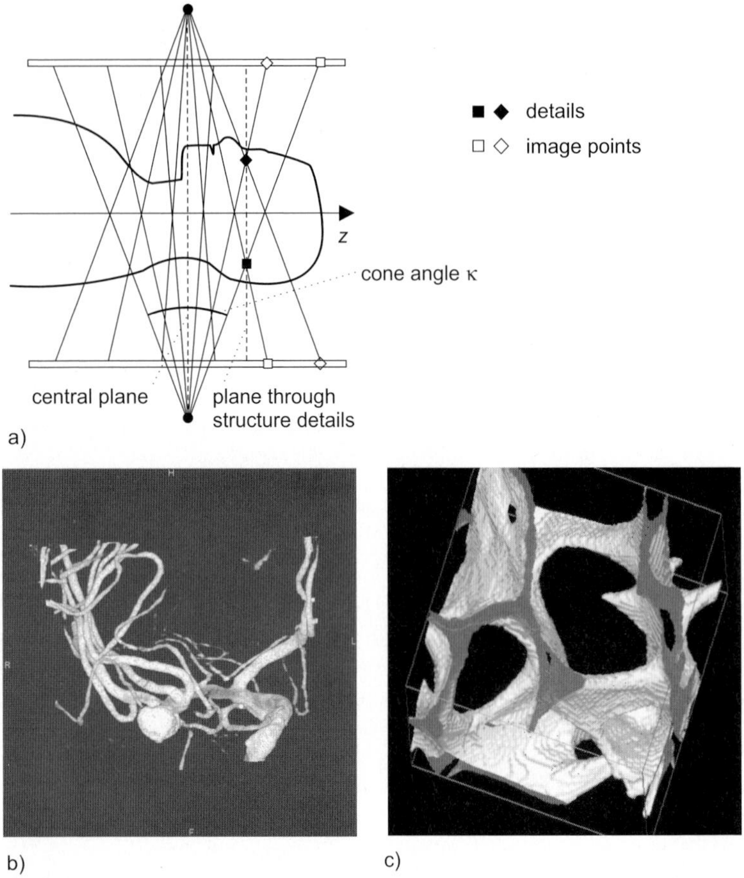

■ ◆ details
□ ◇ image points

cone angle κ

central plane
plane through structure details

a)

b)   c)

Figure 2.12
Cone beam CT. **a)** The larger the cone beam angle, the greater are potential inconsistencies in data. **b)** 3D-angiography with rotating image intensifier. **c)** Micro-CT scans of a bone biopsy with a 1024 × 1024 CCD detector.

9.2.3) and corrections for the increasing contributions from scattered radiation must still be developed to achieve this. This problem constitutes the greatest challenge to physicists and engineers in CT today.

3 Spiral CT

3.1 First Considerations and Efforts

Studies and results on spiral CT were first presented in 1989 at the annual meeting of the Radiological Society of North America (RSNA) [Kalender, 1989; Vock, 1989]. The technical prerequisites had become available with the introduction of the continuously rotating scanners as discussed in the previous chapter. From today's perspective, it appears only logical or even mandatory to introduce spiral CT immediately together with the new scanner technology. However, this was not the case at that time. The development and the introduction of continuously rotating scanners aimed at shorter scan times and at providing improved capabilities for dynamic CT. Spiral CT was not yet known.

The first references to spiral CT can be found in several independent sources. A general patent on spiral scanning does not exist. My own patent request in 1988 was rejected with the statement that the combination of continuous data acquisition and continuous patient transport was already covered by the existing technique of taking survey radiographs (s. section 2.3.1) and that reconstruction algorithms were not patentable. It took time, until the nineties, for the general consensus to develop that algorithms can be patented. A patent by I. Mori [Mori, 1986], the first reference to spiral CT in the patent literature, specified algorithms, but also specified electronic circuits in order to be able to define patent claims. These are hardly useful for the inventor anymore today, since hardware implementations would not be up-to-date and new algorithms are constantly under development. Results on spiral CT from Japan in the English language were first reported in 1993 [Toki, 1993].

W.A. Kalender, Germany, and P. Vock, Switzerland, started in 1988 in the field of spiral CT and were able to present physical measurements and clinical studies on the performance of spiral CT in 1989 [Kalender, 1989; Vock, 1989; Kalender, 1990b]. Parallel to these developments, although also without knowledge of the work carried out elsewhere, Y. Bresler and C.J. Skrabacz of the University of Illinois carried out theoretical studies regarding the spiral scan principle, which were published relatively late [Bresler, 1993]. They characterized their considerations as "intellectually interesting", but of little relevance to practice. This assessment was reinforced by an American CT manufacturer, who also investigated this scan mode, but decided at that time that this was not adequate for general clinical use due to problems which could be expected with image quality [Crawford, 1990].

Such a cautious approach is still understandable today to a certain degree. For sequential CT two basic requirements hold true which cannot be neglected without negative implications for image quality: the object to be scanned, i.e. the patient, may not move during data acquisition, and the scan geometry must be perfectly planar. The consequences are well known if one of these two conditions is violated. If the patient moves or if only inner organs or organ parts move during the scan, motion artifacts result. The same has to be expected if the patient, although cooperative and not moving, is being transported by table motion through the field of measurement (figure 3.1a).

Examples of conflicts with the second requirement – strict adherence to planar scan geometry – were known just the same. Artifacts arise when the focus of the x-ray tube, due to thermal effects or mechanical inaccuracies, does not follow its prescribed path or when the focus and detector do not travel in the same plane. The latter problem exists in particular for EBCT scanners (see section 2.4.1). In general and for the situations described above inconsistent data is generated, since the scanning system does not view exactly the same slice for different angular positions. Such inconsistencies lead to visible artifacts in most cases, as will be discussed further in section 4.1.5.

Spiral CT, however, builds precisely upon violating these two principles: it no longer requires the accepted planar geometry, and it moves the patient during scanning, in classical terms thus constituting a sacrilege. This explains why most of the experts showed more than only minor reservations with respect to the new scan mode. Critics initially termed spiral CT "a method to produce artifacts in CT". Alternatives were suggested, such as the use of moving collimators by GE Medical Systems to combine the advantages of fast volume scanning and planar scan geometry [Toth, 1991]. Also, the technical limitations of the first implementation in 1989 did not allow convincing clinical use: 12 rotations for a maximum of 12 s scan time at maximally 165 mA tube current posed severe limitations. In 1990 the first scanner with a dedicated spiral CT option became available (Siemens SOMATOM PLUS), but it took two more years for spiral CT to become generally acknowledged and accepted as the most important scan mode of future CT scanners.

Reservations with respect to image quality in spiral CT have in the meantime been largely eliminated. The additional computational efforts, various approaches to z-interpolation which provide acceptable images (figure 3.1b), are well known and firmly established today (see chapter 3.3). Some subtle effects may still be observed, but there is no doubt remaining that the advantages of spiral CT prevail, even with respect to image quality. The underlying considerations will be discussed further with respect to

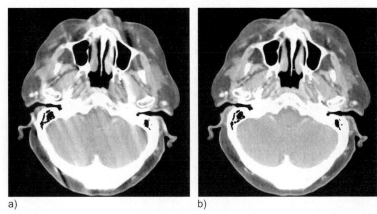

a)   b)

Figure 3.1
Immediate reconstruction of an image from a 360° spiral data segment will produce motion artifacts (**a**). The use of z-interpolation prevents this (**b**) and additionally allows for image reconstruction at arbitrary positions along the z-axis (see below).

image quality in direct comparison with sequential CT in the following chapter. With respect to clinical benefits, there is no doubt that spiral CT offers important advantages and superior performance.

3.2 Scanning Principle and Techniques in Spiral CT

Spiral CT constitutes a volume scanning mode in non-planar geometry with the patient being scanned continuously in space, i.e. along the z-axis, and in time. It represents an alternative to sequential CT, in which volumes are imaged by successively scanning single slices of a stationary object in planar geometry. Spiral scans encompass many rotations of the tube-detector system, while the patient is transported continuously through the gantry. This is typically done at a speed of one to two slice collimations per 360° rotation, i.e. with 1 to 20 mm/s for a 1s scanner and single-row detector with a variable slice width of 1 to 10 mm. For multi-slice systems and sub-second rotation times the table speed can be increased significantly. The transition from a 1s scanner with a single-slice detector to a 0.5s scanner with a four-slice system means a potential increase by a factor of 8.

The focus of the x-ray tube of course continues to travel on a circular path; however, relative to the patient it follows a spiral or helical trajectory (figure 3.2), the origin of the terms spiral and helical used today. Spiral CT and Helical CT can be viewed as synonyms and are both found in the literature [Kalender, 1994a]. The term Spiral CT appears more illustrative – just as 'spiral staircase', 'spiral binder' and other commonly used names are readily understood, as opposed to 'helical staircase' etc. – and is used more frequently. According to authoritative dictionaries which the author and his co-authors consulted before choosing the term spiral in 1989, both terms apply to the given geometry in the English language. (Note: In German mathematical notation 'helical' would be appropriate, but was discarded in order to conform with standard English language usage.)

The choice of parameters in spiral CT corresponds largely to that in sequential CT (Table 2.5). Parameter values may vary, in particular due to possible constraints for spiral scan modes. The maximum available tube currents for spiral scans, for example, are mostly lower than in sequential single-slice scanning in order to prevent overheating of the anode of the x-ray tube during extended scan times (see also figure 2.7). Modern scanners typically allow for scan times up to 100 s and tube currents up to 350 mA. These values are appropriate for many of today's routine clinical applications. But there are new applications, such as multiphasic contrast-enhanced examinations, i.e. dynamic volume scans, and there is an increasing demand for higher isotropic spatial resolution requiring thin-slice techniques, all of which require higher power settings than available today. The alternative to providing higher power, as discussed in several sections, is the more efficient use of the available power by multi-slice scanning.

For spiral scans one additional parameter has to be chosen: the table feed d in mm per 360° rotation. For single-slice scanners with a rotation time of 1 s, which represented the standard in the early nineties, this corresponded exactly to the table speed d' in mm/s. For newer scanners with variable rotation times between 0.5 s and 2.0 s this simple relation no longer applies. More importantly, the number M of simultaneously scanned slices has to be taken into account. The ratio of table feed d to total slice collimation $M \cdot S$ is generally termed the pitch or pitch factor:

$$p = \frac{d}{M \cdot S} \ . \qquad\qquad (3.1)$$

For a four-slice CT scanner, i.e. $M = 4$, with a nominal slice width of $S = 1$ mm and a table feed of $d = 6$ mm per rotation, for example, a pitch of $p = 1.5$ results.

Pitch is a dimensionless quantity. It is of great importance for image quality and dose considerations, as will be illustrated in the following chapters. Misinterpretations and confusion may result if – as recently introduced by some manufacturers – pitch is specified as the ratio d/S. This is not recommended, since the interrelations between pitch and image quality and dose, which are well known and in the meantime well established, are then lost. A ratio $d/S = 3$, which is promoted by one manufacturer as the standard "high quality" scan protocol for its four-slice scanner, obscures the fact that scanning is performed in an overlapping fashion with a pitch of 0.75 and consequently with an increased dose. The situation will become more and more complex as more and different slice numbers M are offered; already today, on a multi-slice CT scanner the alternatives $M = 2$ or $M = 4$ can be

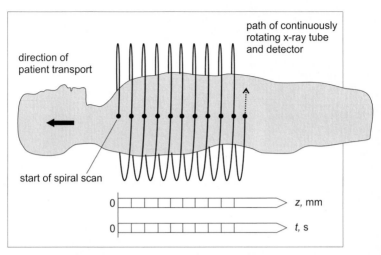

Figure 3.2   Scanning principle of spiral CT [Kalender, 1990b].

chosen. Therefore, the generally accepted definition according to equ. (3.1), which is in agreement with the manufacturers' regulations [IEC, 1999], should be strictly adhered to.

Usually, pitch values between 1 and 2 are chosen. The pitch factor should be larger than 1 to cover a given scan volume as fast as possible and to reduce the dose compared with sequential CT (see section 5.3.2). It should not exceed the value 2, in order to exclude gaps in sampling the object along the z-axis (see below). The choice of the pitch factor is mostly determined by practical considerations – in general by the question of which examination time T (s) is desirable or still acceptable for a given scan range R (mm). The desired table speed $d' = R/T$ (mm/s) then results directly. Taking the selected slice width and pitch factor into account, the table speed actually set is equally given by

$$d' = \frac{p \cdot M \cdot S}{t_{rot}} \; . \tag{3.2}$$

The capability of the most modern scanners to acquire several slices simultaneously ($M > 2$) offers the decisive advantage for the first time of being able to achieve high volume scan speeds coupled with thin slice acquisition ($S < 3$ mm). In addition to technical constraints, the choice of pitch also depends on the available algorithms and parameters for image reconstruction.

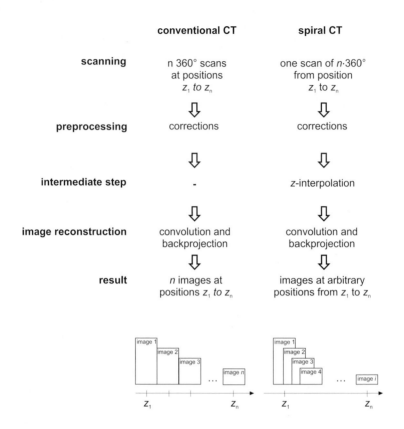

Figure 3.3
Comparison of processing steps from scan to final image for sequential CT (left) and spiral CT (right).

3.3   Image Reconstruction in Spiral CT

The actual image reconstruction in spiral CT is in principle the same as in sequential CT; identical algorithms, convolution kernels and the same hardware are used. However, an additional preprocessing step is required, the so-called z-interpolation. The calculation of images from any 360° spiral data segment leads to artifacts, since different object sections are measured at the start and at the end of any such segment. Such data present inconsistencies (see section 4.1.5); as has to be expected, the resulting artifacts correspond exactly to the motion artifacts known from sequential CT (figure 3.1a).

The z-interpolation is intended to generate a consistent planar data set from the spiral data for an arbitrary image position z_R. Various approaches are available for this purpose. The principal difference relative to sequential CT and a significant advantage at the same time is the inherent possibility of choosing image positions and reconstruction increments (*RI*) freely and retrospectively; the direct coupling between the scan position and the image position, which is unavoidable in sequential CT, no longer exists for spiral CT (figure 3.3). For the image reconstruction itself, the same procedures are again employed, i.e. in practice usually convolution and back-projection. In this last step towards image generation there is no difference between sequential CT and spiral CT.

3.3.1 Basic Approach to *z*-Interpolation (360°LI)

The most straightforward and simplest approach to *z*-interpolation consists of linear interpolation between data measured for a given angular position just before and behind the desired table position z_R, i.e. at a distance d along the *z*-axis or 360° apart along the spiral trajectory, respectively [Kalender, 1990b]. Consequently, we have chosen the term 360°LI for this procedure. The projection $P_z(i, \alpha)$ for projection angle α at a selected position z_R is computed as

$$P_z(i, \alpha) = (1 - w) \cdot P_j(i, \alpha) + w \cdot P_{j+1}(i, \alpha), \tag{3.3}$$

where the interpolation weights (1-*w*) and *w*, respectively, are constant for all channels i of a projection. $P_j(i, \alpha)$ represents the projection in the spiral data set measured in rotation j at position $z_j < z_R$, which was measured closest to the selected position z_R with projection angle α. $P_{j+1}(i, \alpha)$ represents the respective projection at the angle α for the rotation $j+1$. The interpolation weight w is given by

$$w = (z_R - z_j)/d. \tag{3.4}$$

360°LI (figure 3.4a) was the algorithm of choice for the first clinical trials of spiral CT, since it represents a particularly robust approach with respect to image quality. A particular drawback is that slice sensitivity profiles are widened significantly compared with sequential scans, since a data range of $2 \times 360°$ is accessed.

3.3.2 *z*-Interpolation Using Data Rebinning (180°LI)

In the meantime many different spiral algorithms have been developed or proposed. One primary aim has always been to limit the data range accessed for *z*-interpolation in order to keep the slice sensitivity profiles slim (see section 4.2.3). The general approach is to make use of the data redundancy in 360° CT scanning. In any 360° rotation of the x-ray tube, each line integral or projection value is measured twice by two opposing rays, for example the central ray in the a.p. and in the p.a. projection. Using appropriate data sorting or so-called rebinning procedures, this redundancy provides the possibility to determine the projection at an arbitrary angular

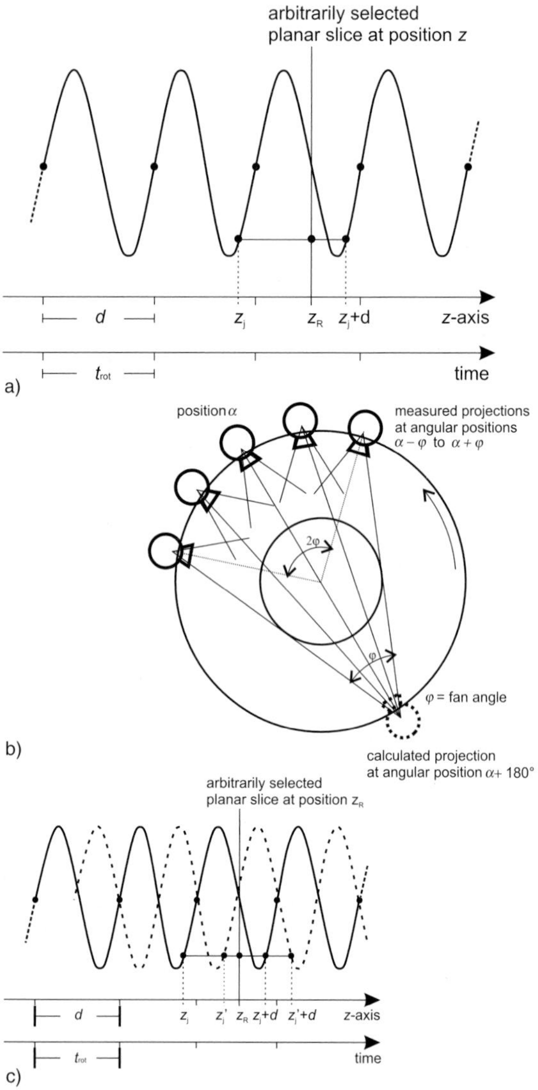

Figure 3.4

Data preprocessing in spiral CT.

a) Linear interpolation between points z_j *and* $z_j + d$ constitutes the simplest approach to estimate values which would have been measured in planar geometry at an arbitrary position z_R (360°LI).

b) For any angular position, projections can be synthesized by rebinning measured values from projections measured in opposing positions.

c) By employing such synthesized spiral data, offset by 180°, data are available for linear interpolation which lie closer to the desired position. Even higher order interpolations can be implemented by using additional measured values.

position from projections measured in opposing directions over an angular range of 2 times the fan angle φ (figure 3.4b). By repeating this for each angular position, a second synthesized spiral can be determined from the measured spiral with both data sets offset to each other by 180°. The synthesized spiral provides the basis for algorithms which use data for interpolation measured only $d/2$, or 180°, apart for the central ray (figure 3.4c). Accordingly, the general term 180° algorithm has been chosen for this approach. The algorithm most widely used today, 180°LI, carries out a linear interpolation accessing a data range of $2 \cdot (180° + \varphi)$ [Polacin, 1992].

A further significant advantage of 180° algorithms is the possibility to extend the table feed d up to two slice thicknesses per rotation, i.e. allowing pitch values of up to 2.0 without any gaps in sampling along the z-direction. Only for p > 2 does the possibility arise that small structural details will not be included within the finite slice collimation for some projection angles. For this reason, pitch factors higher than 2 are generally avoided.

3.3.3 Variations of 180° z-Interpolation Algorithms

It is characteristic of fan beam geometry that, as for partial scans in sequential CT, the angular acquisition range has to be extended to 180° plus the fan angle, while 180° would be sufficient for parallel beam geometry (see section 2.3.2). As a variant which attempts to avoid this extension, the algorithm 180°IX has been proposed [Crawford, 1990]. This accesses a data range of exactly one half rotation before and after the slice position to be reconstructed. Since not all necessary projection values can be determined by interpolation this way, some have to be estimated by extrapolation. This may, however, lead to artifacts in the reconstructed images, arising from the transitions between interpolation and extrapolation or from extrapolation errors. The respective algorithms are termed 180°IX, with X indicating the extrapolation step.

Variations in algorithms may also be due to the type of implementation. The interpolation process, for example, is often implemented in connection with backprojection by a projection-dependent weighting of data. The computation effort for backprojection is increased, in general by a factor of 2, however the explicit interpolation step is omitted. Such a process can be implemented referring to Eq. 3.1 by first backprojecting projection j weighted by $(1-w)$ and thereafter projection j+1 weighted by w in a simple additive manner, with the weight w chosen according to a 360° interpolation. For 180° algorithms the weights are no longer assigned to single rotations, but the procedure is in principle analogous. These weighting algorithms are called 180°WI or 180°WX, respectively, with W indicating the weighted addition in the backprojection process.

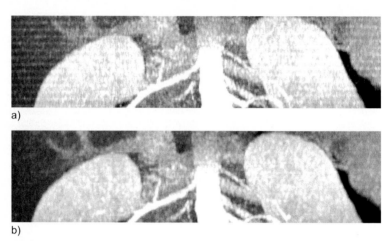

a)

b)

Figure 3.5
The distribution of image noise in Spiral CT depends on the z-position. This may cause horizontal stripe artifacts in MIP displays (**a**), but can be reduced significantly by specially adapted interpolation algorithms (**b**).

In addition, there is also the possibility to employ higher order interpolation algorithms, such as cubic spline functions. For this purpose more than two data points (figure 3.4c) are used to estimate the value which would have been measured in planar geometry. Algorithms of this type are expected to provide improved slice sensitivity profiles, but they will also generate higher image noise [Polacin, 1992]. An analytical prediction of their behavior is in general not possible, since they adapt to the given object. At present, only one manufacturer offers higher order interpolation, however, without exactly specifying the function.

The z-interpolation algorithms presented up to now all have in common that noise levels will be projection-dependent and thereby also z-dependent. As an example it may be noted that for a homogeneous cylindrical object with a constant noise value for all projections, the noise amplitude for projections generated by 360° z-interpolation may vary by up to a factor of $\sqrt{2}$ (see section 4.2.2). The z-dependent noise modulation will increase with increasing distance from the center of rotation and can be observed when browsing through image series or in 3D-displays. For example, the variation in noise amplitude may become visible in maximum intensity projection images (see section 6.3.2) as horizontal stripes originating in the periphery, but not reaching to the center; a horizontal stripe in the opposite direction is displaced in z-direction by a distance $d/2$ (figure 3.5a). Such effects can be reduced by specially designed algorithms. The spiral interpolation algorithm 180°AI reduces the z-dependent noise modulation to a large degree by generating an approximately constant noise level in all synthesized projections. This is achieved by an additional filtering of all

Table 3.1

List and description of z-interpolation algorithms for single-slice spiral CT. 360°LI was used in the first spiral CT systems available; 180°LI and 180°WI represent the algorithms most frequently used today.

Notation	Data range	Short description
360°LI	$2 \cdot 360°$	Linear interpolation between two neighboring rays with identical projection direction and the same angular position (figure 3.4a).
180°LI	$2 \cdot (180° + \varphi)$	Linear interpolation between two neighboring rays with identical projection direction, but opposite angular position (figure 3.4c).
180°IX	$2 \cdot 180°$	Same as 180°LI. X indicates that data missing in the range 180° to 180° + φ are determined by extrapolation.
180°WI	$2 \cdot (180° + \varphi)$	Backprojection of the complete data range with the weighting of projections according to 180°LI; W indicates that interpolation is implemented by weighted backprojection.
180°WX	$2 \cdot 180°$	Backprojection of the complete data range with the weighting of projections, according to 180°IX.
180°HI	$> 2 \cdot (180° + \varphi)$	Higher order interpolation between four neighboring rays of the same projection direction, but different angular positions (figure 3.4c).
180°AI	$2 \cdot (180° + \varphi)$	Additional filtering of projections following spiral interpolation to homogenize noise, for example by using an optimal Wiener filter.
180°CD	$180° + \delta$	ECG-correlated partial scan reconstruction of a data range $180 + \delta$, $\delta < \varphi$
180°CI	$\geq 2 \cdot (180° + \varphi)$	ECG-correlated z-interpolation from data ranges which represent the same cardiac phase.

φ = fan angle

projections after spiral interpolation, providing a noise homogeneity of better than 10 %. MIP displays are thereby improved significantly (figure 3.5b) [Kalender, 1995a].

Special ECG-oriented z-interpolation algorithms have also been developed and meanwhile been set to use successfully [Kachelrieß, 1998b]. These approaches and their generalization to multi-slice spiral CT will be discussed in detail in chapter 3.4.

3.4   Considerations for Multi-slice Spiral CT

3.4.1   z-Interpolation in Multi-slice Spiral CT (180°MLI)

The principle of z-interpolation is independent of the number M of slices acquired simultaneously, as can be seen by direct comparison of figures 3.4c and 3.6a. In each case and for each angular position, the two measured values are selected for z-interpolation from the multitude of data measured closest before and behind the desired z-position. In figure 3.6a the data obtained by rebinning are included; accordingly we speak of 180°MLI algorithms, since all M slices are taken into account for z-interpolation with 180° linear interpolation as described above. Using rebinned data and the two data points closest to the desired position attempts to keep the sensitivity profiles as slim as possible.

3.4.2   z-Filtering in Multi-slice Spiral CT (180°MFI)

The introduction of multi-row detectors and thereby the possibility to acquire several slices per rotation has made it popular and practical to select an effective slice width by choosing a z-filter retrospectively (figure 3.6b). This is possible in principle in single-slice and dual-slice CT systems also. It has become attractive with multi-slice systems, since only here the original data acquisition is carried out routinely with thin slices even for larger volumes. The user can prospectively or retrospectively select the filter width W and potentially the filter function to define the effective slice width and thus also the image noise level and spatial resolution in the z-direction.

Results of z-filtering are illustrated for the example of a lung examination in figure 3.7. The different scanner types in clinical use today permit various approaches and different values of the effective slice thickness; the principle is always the same, however, and corresponds to the procedure of a running mean filtering in image postprocessing, the so-called "sliding thin slab" approach (see chapter 6.2). It is important to realize that the slice thickness can only be increased, but never decreased below the value of the original slice collimation S. A choice of smaller reconstruction increments will in general improve the spatial resolution in the z-direction (see section 4.2.4), since this measure enables finer sampling in the z-direction. The slice collimation itself, i.e. the sampling aperture, remains unchanged.

Here, the principle of z-filtering has been intentionally described in a simple manner, but many variations exist. Approaches have been described by [Taguchi, 1998], [Hu, 1999] and [Flohr, 1999]. In most cases and for most manufacturers, 180°MLI is not directly implemented, since steps and transitions in the data selection from detector slice to detector slice, further

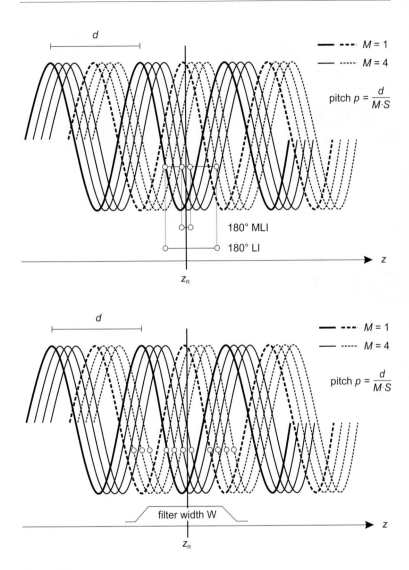

Figure 3.6
For linear z-interpolation in multi-slice spiral CT the two data points closest to the desired image position are used for interpolation (180°MLI) (**a**). In z-filtering (180°MFI) data ranges of variable width are accessed by employing filters of arbitrary form and weighting characteristics (**b**).

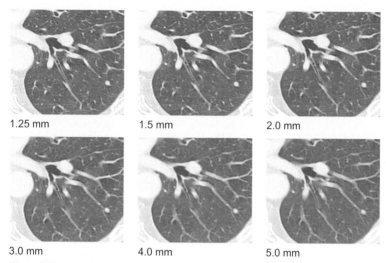

1.25 mm   1.5 mm   2.0 mm

3.0 mm   4.0 mm   5.0 mm

Figure 3.7
z-Filtering allows the generation of images with different effective slice widths and correspondingly altered noise and spatial resolution from a single data set.

complicated by the necessary rebinning processes, may influence image quality negatively. For most CT systems, a variation of 180°MFI with a very small filter width is used to generate soft transitions between various data ranges. For this reason, the minimum effective slice thickness in figure 3.7 is given as 1.25 mm, although 4 × 1 mm collimation has been used. Again, the effective slice width can only be increased to higher values, but never decreased below the colllimated slice width used during acquisition.

3.4.3   ECG-correlated Cardiac Imaging

Due to the permanent motion of the heart during data acquisition, standard image reconstruction often provides images with high artifact content and limited diagnostic use. For typical heart frequencies of 60 to 120 beats per minute (bpm) the duration of one cardiac cycle is in the range of 0.5 to 1.0 seconds, i.e. exactly in the range of the rotation times for modern CT

Figure 3.8 ▶
ECG-correlated z-interpolation.
a) The ECG is recorded synchronously with the CT measurement. The user selects, relative to the R-waves of the ECG, which data ranges are to be accessed for heart phase-oriented image reconstruction.
b) The algorithm 180°MCD represents a partial scan reconstruction using a data range of only slightly more than 180°. Effective scan times are approximately 250 ms to 300 ms for a 0.5 s rotation time.
c) The algorithm 180°MCI implies the usual z-interpolation; however, only data from allowed ranges selected in the ECG will be used. The effective scan time is reduced significantly.

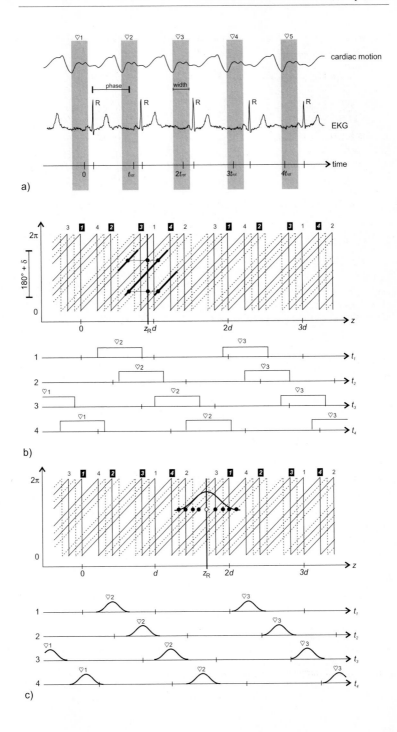

scanners. This often results in an image representing all cardiac phases in a mixed form with varying degrees of artifacts. Algorithms have therefore been developed which use only very short spiral segments or make use of ECG information in z-interpolation to provide images which present the heart in one motion phase only and therefore with greatly reduced effects due to motion. The ECG is recorded simultaneously with the CT measurement in order to be able to correlate cardiac motion with the measured CT data. The user then defines data ranges relative to the ECG which are 'allowed' and can be accessed for reconstruction (figure 3.8a). Such ranges are typically selected relative to the R waves of the ECG signal; for example, the user can center the allowed ranges at 70% of the R-R intervals.

Two classes of algorithms have been developed, 180°CD (cardio delta) and 180°CI (cardio interpolation) and their respective generalizations 180°MCD (multi-slice cardio delta) and 180°MCI (multi-slice cardio interpolation) for single and multi-slice spiral CT, respectively [Kachelrieß, 1998b; Kachelrieß, 2000b]. The algorithms 180°CD and 180°MCD use projection data over a range $180° + \delta$ ($\delta <$ fan angle) for the reconstruction of a partial scan from the spiral data; no z-interpolation is carried out (figure 3.8b). For cardiac imaging δ extends to typically 20°; the effective scan time is then approximately 55% of the rotation time t_{rot}. For a physical rotation time of 0.5 s, for example, effective scan times of about 275 ms result; the limit of 250 ms holds true for the center of rotation. This procedure allows a significant reduction of the motion artifacts. The slice sensitivity profile is defined exactly, and the pitch factor should be chosen as a function of heart frequency (see chapter 7.3). For higher heart frequencies, i.e. when the motion phases of the heart and the diastolic phase in particular are shorter than the effective scan time, there may be some deterioration of the image quality.

The algorithms 180°CI and 180°MCI utilize the information from the simultaneously recorded ECG to ensure that only data acquired during the selected heart phase are used for interpolation (figure 3.8c). They also allow a significant reduction in the effective scan times, since short intervals of the ECG curve are sufficient in most cases; effective scan times of less than 100 ms can be obtained on a 0.5 s scanner for many heart frequencies (see section 7.3). A minor disadvantage is the fact that the slice sensitivity profile is not defined exactly. 180°MCI – labeled as multi-sectoral, biphasic or a similar approach in the manufacturers' implementations – represents the algorithm of choice, in particular when higher heart frequencies are present (see chapter 7.3).

Investigations of cardiac imaging with spiral CT are relatively recent; however, the results are extremely promising. Figure 3.9 serves as an example to illustrate the improvements which subsecond MSCT and ECG-correlated reconstructions offer.

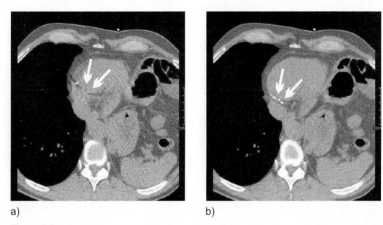

a)   b)

Figure 3.9
Although CT images of the heart obtained with 0.5 s rotation time exhibit a low artifact content, many details, such as the calcified coronary artery, are not displayed sharply in a standard reconstruction (**a**). ECG-correlated z-interpolation improves this situation significantly (**b**).

With the rotation times available today, it is still preferable with respect to image quality to select phases of relatively slow heart motion, i.e. primarily the diastolic phase. It is possible, nevertheless, to generate images for any arbitrary heart phase by continuously shifting the selected ECG interval. Multiplanar and 3D displays of the heart in good quality can then be obtained for successive heart phases, providing the possibility for true 4D imaging of the heart. Acknowledging the expected importance of CT imaging of the heart, this topic will be covered in detail in chapter 7.3; image examples and video clips are also offered on the CD-ROM.

4 Image Quality

The advances in the development of CT image quality were already qualitatively indicated in figure 1.2 and supported with numerical values in table 2.1. Image quality is a concept of central importance for the evaluation of every imaging system. High image quality is with good reason always demanded, but frequently evaluated only subjectively or in a general sense. In this chapter, measured variables and methods for the objective description and quantitative determination of the individual parameters for image quality will be described. In principle, the central issue is always how accurately a system reproduces the object imaged, thus for the case of CT how exactly it represents the object function $O(x,y,z)$, here the three-dimensional attenuation distribution $\mu(x,y,z)$ in the patient. "High fidelity" is expected.

The first question is mostly, how "sharp" is the image. The blurring is described by the point spread function of the system. Mathematically, the image results from the convolution of the object function O with the point spread function PSF. Noise and possibly artifact components, which can prevent the recognition of individual structures, will be superimposed on this image. Furthermore, for every imaging procedure it is necessary to assess the contrast with which the object structures in the image are displayed. For CT, especially the x-ray beam energy, filtration and detector type must be taken into consideration. The respective relationships will be considered here in the form of an energy-dependent contrast factor K. If the individual contributions are known, any image I can be calculated in advance:

$$I(x, y, z) = K \cdot O(x, y, z) * PSF(x, y, z) + \text{noise} + \text{artifacts}. \tag{4.1}$$

Calculations of this kind are actually performed. The computer simulation of the entire measurement and reconstruction process is a valuable and very effective means to clarify the effects of the individual parameters and to introduce suitable development efforts or corrective measures. This also permits the evaluation of very complex and, in part, not yet existing systems, such as cone-beam CT systems and the required new reconstruction procedures which were discussed above.

The purpose of this chapter is to define and explain the underlying variables required for a description of image quality and to illustrate typical values in relation to the apparatus and scan parameters. This will be discussed first for sequential CT, which in text books and standards to date has been treated almost exclusively. The chapter continues with a description of the influences and special considerations of spiral CT and multi-slice spiral CT. The usual, in part legislatively defined requirements for image quality will also be discussed; reference will be made in section 4.3 to the currently valid standards for constancy testing and acceptance testing.

4.1 Variables and Procedures for Sequential CT

4.1.1 CT Values, Contrast and Homogeneity

The CT value scale is defined by the two fixed points 'air = –1000 HU' and 'water = 0 HU' (see section 1.2.4). For every CT scanning unit these fixed points are set using phantom measurements for each high voltage value and each filter and continuously checked as part of maintenance or constancy testing. The goal is to ensure homogeneity, i.e. to maintain a constant CT value for water, over the entire object cross-section The tolerance normally specified as acceptable is up to ±4 HU, which can be checked easily by simple measurements (figure 4.1). Experience shows that this requirement poses no problems for cylindrical water phantoms.

a)   b)

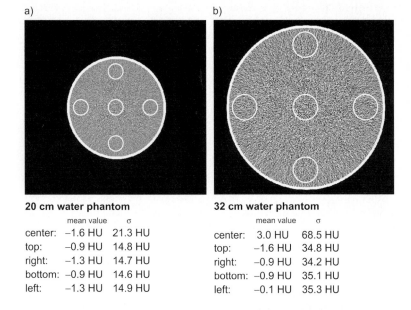

20 cm water phantom

	mean value	σ
center:	–1.6 HU	21.3 HU
top:	–0.9 HU	14.8 HU
right:	–1.3 HU	14.7 HU
bottom:	–0.9 HU	14.6 HU
left:	–1.3 HU	14.9 HU

32 cm water phantom

	mean value	σ
center:	3.0 HU	68.5 HU
top:	–1.6 HU	34.8 HU
right:	–0.9 HU	34.2 HU
bottom:	–0.9 HU	35.1 HU
left:	–0.1 HU	35.3 HU

Figure 4.1
Image homogeneity is usually measured with cylindrical water phantoms.
The CT values for water should not deviate by more than 4 HU from the defined fixed point value of 0 HU for the complete cross-section of phantoms with diameters of 20 cm (**a**) and 32 cm (**b**).

Ensuring the homogeneity of CT values for different object cross-sections is more difficult. For homogeneous phantoms, if only the shape of the cross-section is changed, this is physically possible. A distinguishing characteristic of a good CT scanner is that the CT values for water deviate by only a few HU from the reference value of 0 HU even for oval or elliptical cross-sections. For combinations of materials, on the other hand, this is difficult to achieve.

The CT values of soft tissues (figure 1.9) and therefore their contrast as well, defined as the difference in the CT values of neighboring structures, are only very slightly dependent on the object cross-section. For materials with effective atomic numbers greatly different from that of water, however, the CT values and therefore the contrasts from one scanner to another can vary greatly depending on the particular spectrum and patient diameter. If CT values are to be interpreted quantitatively, such as for the measurement of calcium in bones or in the coronary arteries, a special calibration is required (see chapter 7).

4.1.2   Pixel Noise

Every measured value, including the measurement of attenuation in CT, is in principle subject to an uncertainty. For an ideal system, this error should be purely statistical in origin, i.e. caused by the fluctuations in the number of x-ray quanta registered by the detector. For this reason we also speak of 'quantum noise'. Influences or errors originating in the unit itself – this is the definition of an 'ideal system' – must be negligibly small by comparison. Today's CT scanning systems come very close to achieving this goal, that physically generated quantum noise is the predominant influence.

The noise-related errors in the measurement of the intensity enter into the calculated attenuation values and are further propagated via the image reconstruction, ultimately appearing in the resulting image. Here, these errors can be recognized as image or pixel noise. The pixel noise, designated σ, is determined as the standard deviation of the values I_i from N pixels of a region of interest (ROI) in a homogeneous image section relative to their mean value:

$$\sigma^2 = \frac{1}{N-1} \cdot \sum_{i=1}^{N} (I_i - \bar{I})^2. \tag{4.2}$$

The measurement is normally performed using a water phantom (figure 4.1). The noise value σ increases when the detector registers less x-ray quanta, that is for a high attenuation I_0/I due to strongly absorbing objects, low tube current – scan time products Q (mAs) and a small slice thickness S (mm). Decisive is that the noise changes with the square root of these parameters and not as a linear function:

$$\sigma = f_A \cdot \sqrt{\frac{I_0 / I}{\varepsilon \cdot Q \cdot S}} \ . \qquad (4.3)$$

This means for example that the mAs product – and therefore the dose – must be increased by a factor of 4 in order to reduce the noise by a factor of 2. ε is a measure for the efficiency of the entire system, which the user can not influence significantly. The factor f_A takes account of the effect of the reconstruction algorithm. 'Sharp' high-resolution algorithms increase the noise level, while 'smoothing' contrast-enhancing algorithms reduce the noise level. Table 4.1 indicates noise level values for different reconstruction algorithms.

The influence of quantum noise on the detectability of low-contrast details is illustrated in figure 4.2 for two scans with widely different parameter sets. This example should sharpen the awareness that the noise level, and therefore the contrast differentiation, depends very strongly on the dose and the scanning parameters and that an excessive dose reduction can endanger the diagnosis, in this case especially the detectability of low-contrast structures. Consequently, it is necessary to choose a noise level suitable for the particular indication and patient cross-section. The optimal selection of the scanning and reconstruction parameters is of great importance as will also be discussed in chapter 5.

4.1.3   Spatial Resolution – Resolution at High Contrast

The spatial resolution describes the capability of an imaging system to display fine details separately. It is generally determined for high-contrast structures in order to eliminate the influence of noise on this measurement.

Table 4.1
Typical values for pixel noise in HU for different convolution kernels, object diameters and slice thicknesses, determined by simulation. For the characterization of the convolution kernels typical implementations and names were chosen, which are not necessarily applicable for individual scanning units (primary intensity $2 \cdot 10^5$ quanta per measured data point and mm slice thickness).

Phantom	20 cm water		32 cm water	
Slice thickness	1 mm	10 mm	1 mm	10 mm
Smooth	6.6	2.1	21.2	6.7
Soft	8.2	2.6	26.1	8.2
Standard	9.9	3.1	31.5	10.0
Shepp-Logan	12.3	3.9	39.6	12.5
High	17.9	5.7	57.5	18.1
Ultrahigh	34.9	11.0	112.2	35.4

It is necessary to distinguish between the resolution in the *x*/*y*-scan plane and the resolution in the *z*-direction, or longitudinal body axis, since these two values depend on different factors. The combination of these two values in the form of a '3D-resolution' will be discussed further below in connection with spiral CT, which offers decisive advantages here.

4.1.3.1   Spatial resolution in the scan plane

The resolution in the scan plane depends on the one hand on geometrical variables. This situation can be compared very well with that of conventional radiography; in CT, however, there is the additional influence of the reconstruction algorithm. The decisive geometrical factors influencing the resolution in the scan plane are the focus size, the scan geometry, the detector element spacing and aperture and the movement of the focus during the measurement. These relationships can be viewed in simplified form in the following way, with reference to the variables defined in figure 2.3 and in section 9.1.

As in conventional radiography, the focus size W_F and the detector aperture W_D contribute to image blurring. It is also necessary to consider the geometry of the scanner, since the individual contributions must be weighted appropriately relative to the center of the field of measurement; here R_D and R_F represent the distances from the detector center and the focus, respectively, to the isocenter. This enables us to calculate the corresponding blurring contributions

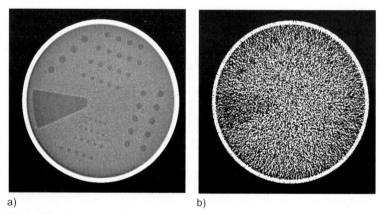

a)   b)

Figure 4.2
The detectability of low-contrast details depends on pixel noise levels as demonstrated here for scans with high dose, e.g. corresponding to a brain examination (**a**), and with very low dose, e.g. corresponding to a bone density measurement (**b**).

$$U_F = \frac{R_D}{R_F + R_D} \cdot W_F \text{ and} \tag{4.4}$$

$$U_D = \frac{R_F}{R_F + R_D} \cdot W_D . \tag{4.5}$$

Since the focus moves continuously and thus also contributes further to the blurring, which is accounted for here in the form of a factor U_B, the blurring induced by the measurement itself is then given by

$$U_{meas.} = \sqrt{U_F^2 + U_D^2 + U_B^2} . \tag{4.6}$$

However, we must also take account of the blurring contribution which arises from the reconstruction algorithm

$$U_A = c_A \cdot a. \tag{4.7}$$

Here, a is the sampling distance (figure 2.3b,c) and c_A a constant representing the algorithm characteristics. The total blurring is then described in this model by

$$U_{total} = \sqrt{U_F^2 + U_D^2 + U_B^2 + U_A^2} . \tag{4.8}$$

The equations above indicate the factors influencing the spatial resolution and also make clear that the user of a given scanning system has only limited possibilities to influence this value. These possibilities consist principally of the choice of convolution kernel, as demonstrated in the examples below. The focus size, sampling distance and, possibly, the detector aperture are set according to the selected scan mode. The focus size can usually be selected directly, but the sampling distance only indirectly, as implied in the individual scan modes and not always recognizable for the user. With some units, it is possible to reduce the size of the detector aperture through the attachment of a high-resolution comb (section 2.2.3), leading to improved resolution but at the same time reducing the geometrical dose efficiency of the detector system.

Direct measurements of the spatial resolution, e.g. with hole patterns and bar tests, as well as indirect methods, such as the calculation of the point spread and modulation transfer function (MTF), are available. Direct measurements are easily performed, easily understood and relatively simple to interpret (figure 4.3a,b). However, their evaluation is also somewhat subjective – according to the choice of the viewing window and personal decision criteria, a series of holes can be assessed as separated, i.e. fully resolved, or as not separated. For technical testing, for example to check whether a system conforms to the manufacturer's specifications, the modulation transfer function is better suited. It is calculated most commonly from the measurement of a thin wire phantom (figure 4.3c). Such a measurement provides the point spread function, which is then subjected to a Fourier transformation to obtain the MTF [Rossmann, 1969]. The MTF is

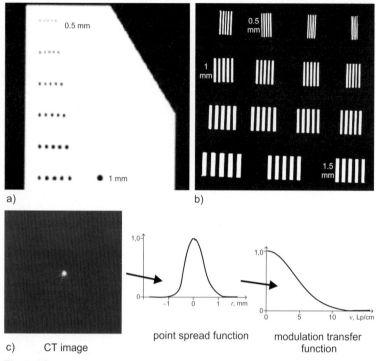

Figure 4.3
Various resolution tests and the resulting images.
a) Drilled hole pattern. **b)** Bar pattern. **c)** Wire phantom for measurement of the point spread function and calculation of the modulation transfer function.

an objective measure of the contrast with which the individual frequencies (object modulations, measured in line pairs per cm, Lp/cm) are reproduced by the particular imaging system.

The determination of the MTF, while requiring computer calculations, yields information about the entire frequency range and offers the advantage that it yields objective and quantitative information. In addition to measurements on thin wire phantoms to determine the point spread function, edge phantoms or periodic square wave patterns (figure 4.3b) are also available for the determination of edge response functions and rectangular MTFs, respectively, followed by calculation of the MTFs. It should be pointed out, however, that these latter methods are prone to errors and disturbances, so that wire phantom measurements are viewed as today's standard method.

Spatial resolution is mostly specified in terms of the frequency for a given percent value of the MTF. The spatial resolution obtainable for a given

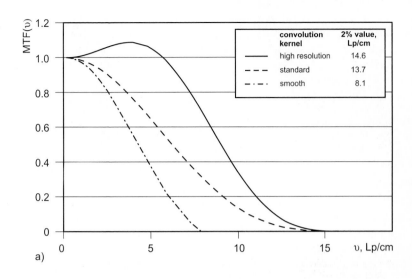

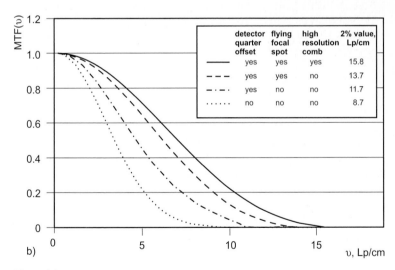

Figure 4.4
Modulation transfer functions for various convolution kernels **(a)** and scan modes **(b)**.

system is often specified according to the 2% value of the MTF; i.e., the frequency at which the contrast has dropped to 2% of the maximum value obtained at 0 Lp/cm. Systems on today's market attain resolutions of up to 20 Lp/cm or more. It is clear that spatial resolution depends on the choice of convolution kernel. The maximum obtainable resolution for a scanning system is calculated using 'sharp' kernels (figure 4.4a). This also considerably increases the pixel noise (table 4.1), leading to the increased occurrence of structured noise and streak artifacts. Reconstructions with kernels designated by such terms as 'ultrahigh resolution' can therefore be recommended only with high contrast objects and a wide viewing window. Reconstructions with standard and 'smoothing' kernels will reduce the maximum obtainable resolution, but also noise and artifacts, improving the low-contrast detectability.

The influence of different scan modes can be most effectively assessed by MTF determinations. Thus, for example, the expected positive effects of the quarter detector offset, flying focal spot and high-resolution comb on spatial resolution can be clearly demonstrated; to enable better comparisons, the standard convolution kernel has been used here in all cases (figure 4.4b). For the combination of the high-resolution scan mode and the high-resolution convolution kernel, the 2% value of the MTF exceeds 20 Lp/cm for the system represented in figure 4.4.

4.1.3.2   Influence of the image matrix

Equation (4.8) does not consider the matrix size, that is the size of the individual pixels. Nevertheless, this is another, in practice, relevant influence on the spatial resolution in the scan plane. The limiting resolution, referred to in all technical specifications, is always determined using a reconstruction with a large zoom factor in order to exclude the influence of the image matrix. For zoom factors of five or greater, this is certainly the case, but for the routinely used values between 1.2 and 2.0 this is mostly not so. These relationships are relatively easy to assess.

During the scan the particular field of measurement (FOM) with diameter D_{FOM} is acquired completely and – depending on the selected zoom factor ZF – is displayed either in its entirety ($ZF = 1$) or only a section thereof ($ZF > 1$) in a field of view (FOV) with a diameter D_{FOV}:

$$D_{\text{FOV}} = \frac{D_{\text{FOM}}}{ZF}.$$ (4.9)

A square matrix of the size $N_{\text{pixel}} \times N_{\text{pixel}}$ is normally calculated. The resulting pixel size is then

$$W_{\text{pixel}} = \frac{D_{\text{FOV}}}{N_{\text{pixel}}}.$$ (4.10)

Figure 4.5 ▶
When using low zoom factors spatial resolution may be limited by the matrix size or pixel size. Reconstruction with the zoom factor 1.5 and magnification by a factor 5 does not provide the resolution achieved by reconstruction with the zoom factor 7.5. This is evident both in scans of a resolution test (**a**) and in clinical images (**b**).

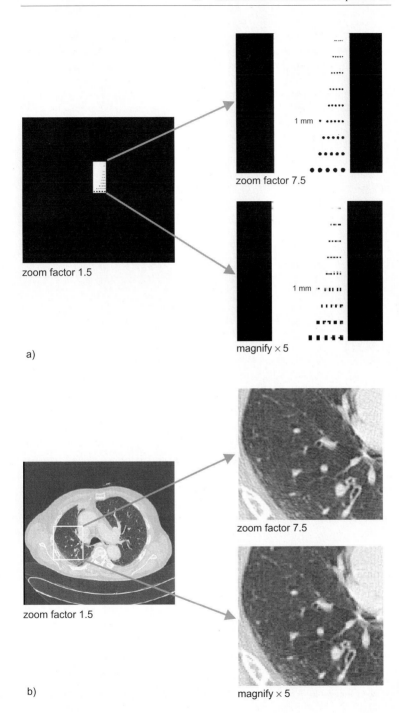

zoom factor 7.5

1 mm

zoom factor 1.5

magnify × 5

a)

zoom factor 7.5

zoom factor 1.5

b)

magnify × 5

Today, a matrix of 512×512 pixels, with a field of measurement of approximately 50 cm, is commonly calculated in CT. Using an exact value of $D_{FOM} = 51.2$ cm, for example, the resulting pixel sizes are 1.0, 0.5 and 0.2 mm corresponding to zoom factors of 1, 2 and 5, respectively. Thus, for example, if typical resolution values of 5–10 Lp/cm are required or expected, corresponding to detail sizes of 0.5–1 mm, the zoom factors of 1.2 to 1.8 usually employed for lung scans are too low.

A negative influence of the image matrix is largely excluded when the pixel size is smaller than the diameter of the smallest resolvable detail d_{min} by a factor of two or more (Nyquist condition). In general, this condition can be expressed as:

$$W_{pixel} \leqslant 0.5 \cdot d_{min} . \tag{4.11}$$

For the assumed field of measurement with a diameter of 51.2 cm and a matrix of 512×512, for a given resolution value, specified as a detail diameter in mm, a zoom factor of at least

$$ZF > \frac{2 \text{ mm}}{d_{min}} \tag{4.12}$$

must be selected. I.e., for example, a zoom factor of 4 or larger has to be selected if details of 0.5 mm are to be resolved. A subsequent enlargement of the image, frequently offered as a "magnify" function or as a "magnifying glass", while it provides a finer display matrix and gives a more pleasant image, cannot compensate for the loss of resolution resulting from an insufficient reconstruction matrix (figure 4.5).

4.1.3.3   Slice sensitivity profiles

The slice sensitivity profile (SSP) represents the system's response perpendicular to the scan plane, comparable with the point spread function in the scan plane. It specifies with which signal contribution an infinitesimally small object at a given position on the z-axis is represented in the image. Ideally, a small object within the slice should yield 100 % signal and objects outside the slice should yield 0 % signal. Two principal approaches are mostly used for the measurement of the slice sensitivity profile, the so-called ramp and delta phantoms.

Ramp phantoms are usually implemented in the form of thin strips, such as aluminum with a thickness of 0.1 mm, attached at a particular angle with respect to the z-axis. In this way, in sequential CT the slice profile can be measured quickly and without problems; the profile is determined directly in the image and then evaluated (figure 4.6a). For spiral CT, however, ramps do not produce reliable results [Polacin, 1994].

Delta phantoms, on the other hand, do not fill out the entire slice as for ramp phantoms, but instead represent a delta impulse, i.e. an impulse

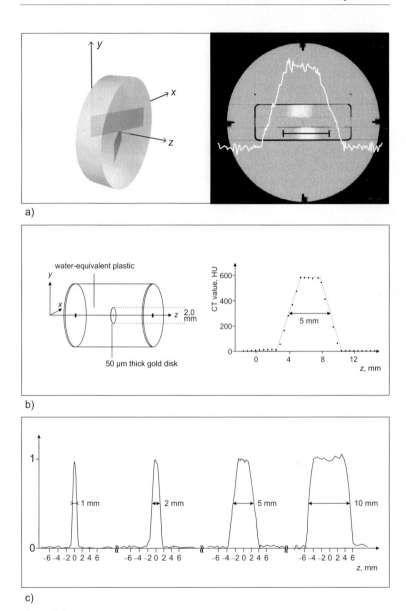

a)

b)

c)

Figure 4.6
For measurements of slice sensitivity profiles ramp **(a)** and impulse or delta phantoms **(b)** are generally available. Ramps are used predominantly in sequential CT, as for the examples shown in **(c)**, while delta phantoms are required for spiral CT.

which ideally has an infinitesimally small extent in the z-direction. For this method, small thin platelets or tiny spheres of high density and with a high atomic number are suited to a good approximation. As an example, figure 4.6b depicts a gold platelet of 50 μm thickness with a diameter of 2 mm. Delta phantoms are ideally suited for spiral CT, since they are continuously moved with the scan along the z-axis. Their use is also possible in sequential CT and provides good results, but is cumbersome since it requires a large number of individual measurements in order to sample the entire profile.

The scanned section is generally characterized by the full width of the profile at 50 % of its maximum value (Full Width at Half Maximum, *FWHM*). This value is designated as the nominal slice thickness and is also defined in this way in the usual regulations. The FWHM, however, gives no information about whether the profile approximates the ideal shape of a rectangle or deviates substantially from this shape. Slice profiles for standard CT are good approximations to the ideal rectangular shape for thick slices (figure 4.6c). On the other hand, for thin slices it is necessary to insert collimators close to the detector in order to obtain this shape. Due to dose considerations, however (see section 5.2), this is seldom done. In spiral CT the SSPs are smoothed further, as will be shown below. For the same full width at half maximum it is therefore possible to encounter approximately rectangular, triangular or Gauss-shaped profiles.

The shape of the SSP has a very considerable influence on the imaging of smaller object details, as illustrated schematically in figure 4.7a. The contrast of an object, which is smaller than the slice thickness and located only partly in the scanned slice, is reduced according to the extent to which it is positioned in the particular volume element. This linear partial volume effect is unavoidable, but can be reduced or eliminated altogether by the selection of thinner slices. More important is the discrimination between neighboring slices, which depends to a large extent on the shape of the profile. For an ideal rectangular profile, only those structures contribute to the signal which are actually located within the nominal slice thickness S. On the other hand, for non-ideal profiles structures located outside of the nominal slice thickness also contribute to the image. Even a minimal tail of the profile can permit high-contrast details to still produce visible contributions to the image, which are superimposed onto low-contrast structures and can mask these to the point of unrecognizability. As an example, this phenomenon can be observed in the vicinity of the base of the skull. The shape of the sensitivity profile thus plays an important role for excluding crosstalk between neighboring slices. This can be seen clearly in the example of figure 4.7a.

Since the shape of the profile is not represented in the *FWHM* value, that is in the specification of the nominal slice width S, there is a need for additional figures of merit to characterize this. Linear variables (figure 4.7b),

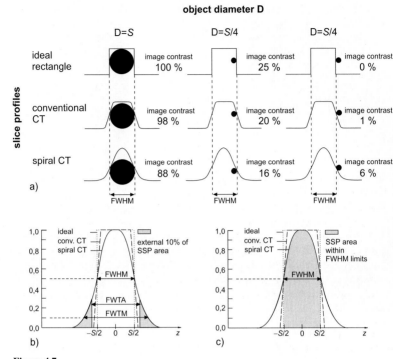

Figure 4.7
Significance of and descriptors for the shapes of SSPs (see text).
a) Influence of SSP shape on imaging small objects.
b), c) Specifying the full width at half maximum does not suffice to characterize the SSP's quality. Additional figures of merit and indices are required.

such as the profile width at 10 % of the maximum value (Full Width at one Tenth of Maximum, *FWTM*) and the width of the profile at a height which includes 90 % of the area under the profile and excludes 10 % (Full Width at Tenth Area, *FWTA*) [Polacin, 1992] have been proposed. Another possibility is in the form of an integral measure (figure 4.7c) and is called the slice profile quality index (*SPQI*) [Kalender, 1995a]:

$$SPQI = \frac{\text{Area bounded by nominal slice width}}{\text{Area of ideal profile}} \cdot 100\%. \qquad (4.13)$$

The *SPQI* therefore specifies how closely a profile approximates the ideal value of 100 %, which corresponds to the ideal rectangular shape. Examples of values for the proposed figures of merit will be presented in connection with spiral CT in table 4.4.

4.1.3.4 Spatial resolution along the z-axis

The resolution along the z-axis has seldom been measured in CT or in other slice imaging modalities. This parameter has been largely ignored; in most cases, it would only have documented the flagrant disparity between the resolution in the x/y-scan plane and the resolution in the z-direction. Until now, estimates of the z-resolution have been mostly limited to specifying the slice thickness. In view of the increasing importance and availability of volume examinations and 3D representations, however, measurements of z-axis resolution are increasingly gaining in importance.

Whereas several established methods are available for the measurement of the resolution in the scan plane (figure 4.3) and the corresponding values are also given by the manufacturers for all CT scanning systems, for the measurement of the spatial resolution in the direction of table feed there are no established methods. Here as well, it is possible to call upon several methods. Of these, test patterns can be recommended on the basis of their simplicity of use and their ease of understanding. Drilled hole tests can be positioned in the direction of table feed just as well as in the scan plane. After the scan and the image reconstruction, a multiplanar reformatting (MPR, see section 6.2) must follow in the x/z- or y/z-plane, which can then be directly evaluated. An example of this will be shown in section 4.2.4 (figure 4.14).

Alternatively, it is also possible to calculate the MTF. As for the scan plane, this is given in the z-direction as well by the Fourier transformation of the point spread function, that is here of the slice sensitivity profile. In practice problems arise due to inevitable slight errors in the measurement of the SSPs, which however strongly influence the calculation of the MTF, especially the determination of the 2 % value or the cut-off frequency [Süß, 1995]. In order to actually obtain the resolution values defined by the MTF, it is necessary to sample with sufficient precision along the z-axis. This means that the increment between images should be less than one fifth of the slice thickness. In sequential CT this is not practical, which is why we recommend simple tests, such as drilled hole patterns. For spiral CT, on the other hand, with the calculation of overlapping images, MTF measurements can be performed more easily.

4.1.3.5 High-resolution CT

The term high-resolution CT derives from about the year 1980 and referred primarily to the introduction of new methods of image reconstruction. Whereas the improvement which the quarter detector offset (see section 2.2.1) brought in the sampling rate had been employed until then exclusively for the reduction of artifacts, for the first time methods were now used which, by way of a resorting of the data from oppositely positioned projections, the so-called rebinning (see section 3.3.2), generated projections with twice the number of measured values. This halved the sampling distance and, as expected from equ. (4.8), led to higher resolution. The third dimension was however still disregarded. Thin slice techniques were introduced only somewhat later; the first work with 1 mm slices was carried out in 1985. While the term high-resolution CT thus originally referred only to a specific reconstruction method, today we understand this to mean an entire bundle of measures, which must all be matched to one another. To these belong in particular the selection of a corresponding scan mode with thin slices and image reconstruction at small reconstruction increments with a high-resolution convolution kernel and a high zoom factor.

4.1.4   Contrast Resolution – Resolution at Low Contrast

Low-contrast resolution, i.e. in general the capability to detect details at low contrast, represents one of the most important tasks of all sectional imaging methods. This was in fact the superior figure of merit which helped CT to achieve its rapid breakthrough in the early seventies. In practice, this is largely a question of the soft tissue contrasts which result from differences in density and depend only weakly on the energy of the x-ray quanta. The low-contrast detectability is determined primarily by the noise level in the image (figure 4.2) and consequently by the influences on noise discussed above. While measurements of the pixel noise σ are very simple to perform, the specification of contrast resolution is difficult and always a matter of subjective assessment. On the basis of phantom scans (figure 4.8), an observer must decide which series of bore holes can be recognized as separated or as not separated. As a result of this subjective type of evaluation, it is not always possible to exactly reproduce the contrast resolution specified for a scanning system, just as for the evaluation of artifacts. To make matters more difficult, the different phantoms to be found on the market give rise to different evaluations of the same system, since these results are in part dependent on the energy spectrum and the temperature of the phantom material [Süß, 1999]. There is therefore a need for the standardization of low-contrast measurements.

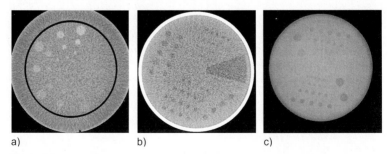

a)   b)   c)

Figure 4.8
Various phantoms are available for the measurement of low-contrast resolution, such as the Catphan (**a**), the ATS phantom (**b**) and the QRM LowC phantom (**c**). However, these may give contradictory results [Süß, 1999].

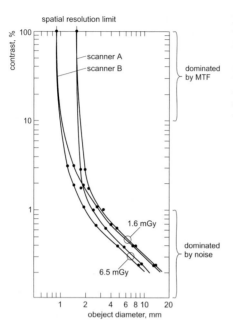

Figure 4.9
Contrast-detail diagrams reflect the influence of quantum noise and spatial resolution on the detectability of object details. For structures with contrast and diameter above or to the right of the respective curve, adequate resolution can be expected [Cohen, 1979].

Contrast resolution is determined not only by the signal-to-noise ratio (SNR), i.e. the quotient of the difference in CT values to the pixel noise level, but by the spatial resolution of the system as well, since low-contrast structures of different sizes can occur. This relationship is made clear by contrast-detail curves. The limit value of curves for small objects corresponds to the spatial resolution limit and results from the system parameters discussed in section 4.1.3. These values are obtained only for high contrasts, in keeping with the definition of spatial resolution. The contrast-dependent resolution values for larger objects are dependent on the noise level and therefore on the dose level and the dose efficiency of the system. This is expressed in the right section of the curves. Due to the statistical nature of noise and the subjective criteria for recognition, a large uncertainty results for the determination of the individual measured values. The region of transition between the two sections of the curve indicates that, for the same noise level, a system with a higher spatial resolution offers a higher contrast resolution for small lesions (figure 4.9).

4.1.5   Artifacts

Independently of the image quality parameters already discussed, which we can evaluate objectively and quantitatively to a large degree, we must also evaluate the image with regard to the question of whether it faithfully reproduces the actual object. The imaging system may produce artificial structures which deviate from reality, that is artifacts (lat.: arte factum). A decision on what is correct and what is not correct, what is imaged correctly or artificially produced, is not always an easy matter in patient acquisitions and requires considerable experience on the part of the examiner, as well as a proper knowledge of the system's artifact behavior. Fortunately, CT has in the meantime overcome a number of 'infant diseases' of a technical character, such as the dropout of individual measured values or differences in the sensitivities of the individual detector channels, which lead to streak or ring artifacts (figure 4.10a). Nevertheless, there remain certain artifacts which are caused by the physical nature of CT, artifacts of which the examiner must also be aware and which frequently can be controlled only through a suitable choice of scan parameters.

Important causes of artifacts are patient movement, beam hardening, scattered radiation, partial volume effects, metallic implants, sampling errors and exceeding the limits of the field of measurement. A general consideration of how artifacts arise can be seen for the example of patient movement. With CT, patient movement leads not only to local blurring of the contours, as is known from radiography, but also to disturbances throughout the entire image (figure 4.10b). This is a consequence of the principle of image reconstruction in CT. As was illustrated in figure 1.7, during the backprojection every detail contributes information to each pixel. Balancing out the undesired contributions outside of the pixel in question is only possible if the object does not move or change during the acquisition, in other words if the projection data from the different directions consistently describe the same object function $O(x,y,z)$. Inconsistencies in the data acquired therefore always cause disturbances throughout the entire image. But these disturbances are not necessarily immediately apparent, since such disturbances sometimes express themselves in the form of falsified CT values only, as is often the case with errors caused by beam hardening (see below). As a rule, it can be said that image disturbances are most pronounced close to the site of their origin, but that they can still affect the image at greater distances from this site.

Whereas motion artifacts are generally known and can be intuitively understood, the origin and explanation of other types of artifacts is more complex. Such artifacts will be shown here only by way of example, with brief explanations. Beam hardening is seen in CT images mostly as dark zones or streaks between bone structures. A typical case is for acquisitions in the vicinity of the base of the skull, between the petrous bones; the term "Hounsfield bar" (figure 4.10c) was coined to describe this phenomenon. Beam hardening artifacts result because the broad polychromatic spectrum of the x-radiation is attenuated differently, depending on the energy of the radiation, the object type and projection direction, and consequently causes variable increases in the mean energy of the spectrum when encountering thicker objects and especially bony structures. This also means that μ, as a function of the varying mean energies, varies with the projection direction;

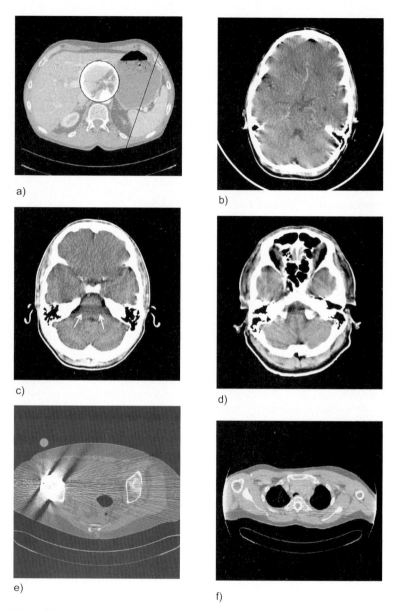

a)

b)

c)

d)

e)

f)

Figure 4.10
Typical examples for artifacts in CT images which may result from failures of the detector
electronics **(a)**, patient motion **(b)**, beam hardening **(c)**, partial volume effects **(d)**, metallic
implants **(e)** or the patient exceeding the field of measurement **(f)**.

i.e., inconsistent data arise. This mostly causes dark 'hypodense' zones in the image. For soft tissues, which resemble water in their beam hardening characteristics, these effects can be corrected, but a simultaneous correction for water, bone and contrast medium is possible only with considerable effort. Some manufacturers offer a specific bone correction for their brain scans for that purpose. The user has only very limited possibilities for influencing this type of artifact.

Partial volume artifacts occur when high-contrast structures extend only partly into the slice examined, since each detector element inevitably averages the radiation intensities in z-direction for that structure and the surroundings instead of the attenuation values to be determined, intrinsically ignoring the logarithmic relationship between intensities and attenuation values. For this reason, this type of artifact is often characterized as the non-linear partial volume artifact. Here again, the posterior cranial fossa is the most critical region (figure 4.10d). Primarily streak-shaped, dark and light, artifacts are produced. The only adequate measure against partial volume effects is to use thin slices. If this causes an excessive increase in the noise level, several thin slices can be summed, as a result of which the image of a thicker slice with a lower noise level, but without the scan-induced artifacts, results. This possibility is available on some scanners as a 'Volume Artifact Reduction' (VAR) technique (see also figure 4.16). Partial volume effects can occur not only in the z-direction but in the scan plane too. In such cases, we generally speak of sampling artifacts; they occur primarily at transitions with very high contrast, such as with metallic objects.

With metallic implants, beam hardening and partial volume artifacts are intensified and can completely extinguish the image contents in the vicinity of the metallic object, leaving only disturbing noise structures (figure 4.10e). Fine streaks which still disturb the image at a larger distance from the origin of the disturbance indicate that, as an additional effect, the sampling procedure is too coarse for the sharp metal-tissue transitions. Together with reducing the slice thickness and selecting the highest kVp value, it can only be recommended with metallic implants that the slice orientation be so selected as to exclude the implant as well as possible from the scanned section. This is often possible for acquisitions in the region of the jaw. Approaches for the reduction of metal-induced artifacts have been provided [Kalender, 1987b], however these are no longer available as a product. New approaches are currently under investigation at the IMP, with the particular goal of eliminating disturbing noise structures [Kachelrieß, 1998a].

Artifacts can also occur if parts of the patient or other objects are in fact in the gantry, but are positioned outside of the field of measurement. Exceeding the limits of the field of measurement leads to hyperdense areas near the exceeding peripheral regions, which are often tolerable (figure 4.10f). However, if discontinuities in contrast are also found in this outer region, such as the patient's arms or ECG cables, streak artifacts can result, which affect the entire image. This type of artifact can be reduced to a large extent by special correction measures [Ohnesorge, 2000].

Image artifacts can frequently be ascribed to the interaction of several of the causes referred to above. The Hounsfield bar, for example, usually includes streaks which result from partial volume effects. For this reason, an analysis is not always easy or unequivocal. In spite of the many causes of artifacts, however, not all of which can be dealt with here for reasons of space, it must be recognized that modern CT, with its highly developed technology, short scan times and with the trend to thinner slices, is now able to routinely produce images which are largely artifact-free.

4.2   Variables and Procedures for Spiral CT

4.2.1   General Considerations

Although all new CT scanning systems have been optimized for spiral CT, especially with regard to x-ray and computer power, it is still possible to acquire single slice scans. This means that the same system components, frequently with the same selection of parameters, are utilized. What are the implications of this for comparing the image quality of sequential CT with that of spiral CT?

It can be expected that the image quality in spiral CT is in every respect comparable with that of sequential CT. Furthermore, the same interrelationships must apply as for a conventional scan of a single slice. For example, the spatial resolution in the x/y-scan plane must be identical, provided that the same reconstruction parameters are selected, because the geometry of the scanner, the number of and separation between the detector elements, the number of projections processed per image etc. all remain unchanged. And the spatial resolution in the x/y-scan plane is in fact found to be unchanged, as can be verified at any time. The quality of the x-ray spectrum is likewise independent of the scan mode. The CT values for any arbitrary object must therefore agree for both cases, and this also means that the contrast remains unchanged. The special case of objects having a diameter smaller than or approximately equal to the slice thickness and for which differences in the contrast behavior that depend on the shape of the slice sensitivity profile can occur will be analyzed in detail below.

Differences can occur in image quality due to the additional z-interpolation processing step in spiral CT in regard to the following parameters:

- pixel noise,
- slice sensitivity profiles,

- resolution in the z-direction and

- artifact behavior

With respect to the pixel noise and the slice sensitivity profile, differences must be expected and in fact do occur. It follows immediately from this that the resolution in the z-direction is also affected. Moreover, subtle differences in artifact behavior can also occur, which are observed increasingly towards the periphery of the field of measurement. The differences in the parameters referred to will be explained in the following, which also considers the dependence on the z-interpolation algorithm employed.

4.2.2 Pixel Noise

In spiral CT, the pixel noise depends on the system used and on the scanning and reconstruction parameters in the same way as for sequential CT. However, it is also influenced by the selection of the z-interpolation algorithm. A direct comparison with sequential CT scans of course assumes that the slice collimation, tube voltage and current and the reconstruction parameters are all identical. Under these assumptions the noise behavior using a linear 360° interpolation can be determined easily relative to a single-slice scan.

σ_0 here designates the standard deviation of the measured projection values and w the interpolation weighting function according to equ. (3.4). In accordance with the rules of error propagation, for linear interpolation the standard deviation of the interpolated data is then given by:

$$\sigma^2 = w^2 \cdot \sigma^2_0 + (1-w)^2 \cdot \sigma^2_0 . \tag{4.14}$$

The variance σ^2 of each measured value determined in this way will be reduced relative to σ_0 in accordance with the weighting function w by a factor which lies between 0.5 and 1.0. For a 360° rotation, i.e. integrating over all weighting factors w, we obtain

$$\sigma^2 = \int_0^1 [w^2 \cdot \sigma^2_0 + (1-w)^2 \cdot \sigma^2_0] \, dw = \frac{2}{3} \sigma_0^2 \tag{4.15}$$

and therefore

$$\sigma = \sqrt{2/3} \cdot \sigma_0 \cong 0.82 \cdot \sigma_0. \tag{4.16}$$

This tells us that we can expect a reduction in the pixel noise by a factor of about 0.82. A reduction is already to be expected due to the fact that, for the reconstruction of any image, data are taken from a range $2 \cdot 360°$ instead of only 360° as for sequential CT.

With the use of 180°LI algorithms, the data used are taken from a smaller angular range than with the 360° interpolation, and the noise values should therefore be higher. For a pixel located at the center of rotation, data are processed over $2 \cdot 180°$. An increase in noise by a factor of $\sqrt{2}$ compared

Table 4.2
Pixel noise in spiral CT relative to sequential scans ($d = 0$ mm/360°) with otherwise identical parameters [Kalender, 1991b].

a) Comparison of theoretically predicted and measured values of relative pixel noise for different algorithms

Interpolation algorithm	Theoretical value	Measured value
360°LI	0.82	0.83
180°LI	1.13	1.12
180°HI	–	1.29

b) Dependence on table feed d

d	Pitch	Pixel noise	
mm/360°	–	HU	relative units
0	0	4.34	1.0
2	0.4	3.61	0.83
5	1.0	3.60	0.83
8	1.8	3.58	0.82
10	2.0	3.61	0.83

with the 360°LI algorithm then results. The ratio of the standard deviations of the 180°LI spiral-interpolated to the sequential CT images should then be $\sqrt{2} \cdot \sqrt{2/3}$. For pixels at a greater distance from the isocenter, the range from which projection data are processed increases to $2 \cdot (180° + \varphi)$; this should become apparent in the form of a slight noise reduction. Following this analysis, we can then expect relative noise values of about 1.15. It is also to be expected that the noise level does not depend on the pitch factor, since the number of measured data processed and the dose setting are defined independently of the table speed. For higher order interpolation methods it is usually not possible to predict the noise behavior, since this depends on the structure of the object examined and the type of algorithm. In general, though, a slight increase in the pixel noise can be expected compared with 180°LI algorithms.

These fundamental considerations can be verified by phantom investigations, with regard to both noise values (table 4.3a) and to the fact that the noise level is independent of the table advance per gantry rotation, that is of the pitch factor (table 4.3b). The noise behavior observed with spiral CT thus becomes understandable, and the differences in the noise level compared with sequential CT are no greater than 20 %. Inhomogeneities in the distribution of the pixel noise at the periphery of the field of measurement which change with the z-position of the reconstructed slice will be discussed in section 4.2.5.

4.2.3   Slice Sensitivity Profiles

It is possible to calculate the behavior of the slice sensitivity profile in spiral CT beforehand also, provided that the original profile, i.e. the SSP of a sequential CT scan, is known. The theoretical considerations and the mathematical derivation can be found in [Kalender, 1991b]. The result is that for spiral CT the slice sensitivity profile is given by the convolution of the original profile with a function of the table movement (figure 4.11a). For linear interpolation, this function corresponds to a triangular motion function with a base length equal to the table feed d (180°LI) or $2d$ (360°LI), respectively. For $d = 0$ (no table advance) the table movement function reduces to the delta function, with the result that the slice profile then remains unchanged. This can be seen physically as the trivial fact that spiral CT without table advance is identical with sequential CT.

For the measurement of slice sensitivity profiles in spiral CT delta phantoms are employed. The agreement between the measured results and the expected results is convincing [Kalender, 1990b; Kalender, 1991b]. Figure 4.11a right shows an example of this. The standard method of employing ramp phantoms, on the other hand, yields inconsistent results and frequently distorted profiles. This problem has been analyzed and the complete explanation can be found in [Polacin, 1994]. The spiral scanning technique can produce artifacts if objects with very high contrast are inclined against the scan slice. In this respect ramp phantoms, which are usually a thin metal sheet with an angle of inclination of 10° to 45°, represent the most unfavorable situation conceivable.

4.2.3.1   Influence of z-interpolation algorithms and pitch factor

As was discussed above, the type of z-interpolation and the pitch factor determine the width of the data range accessed for each image. 360°LI requires two complete revolutions and 180°LI only $2 \cdot (180° + \varphi)$ (see table 3.3). Taking the table feed d in mm per 360° rotation into account, the scan range in mm results which contributes to the particular image. The resulting sensitivity profiles are shown in figure 4.11b, c. As expected, the deviation from the ideal rectangular-shaped SSP increases with the pitch factor, for 360°LI more strongly than for 180°LI. This does not necessarily affect the half-value width; for a pitch of 1 and 180°LI, for example, the same FWHM value is found as in sequential CT. The figures of merit described in section 4.1.3.3 are a better basis for differentiating here (table 4.4). The results for 360°LI at $p = 1$ and 180°LI at $p = 2$ match, as must be expected theoretically, since the table motion functions are identical for these settings.

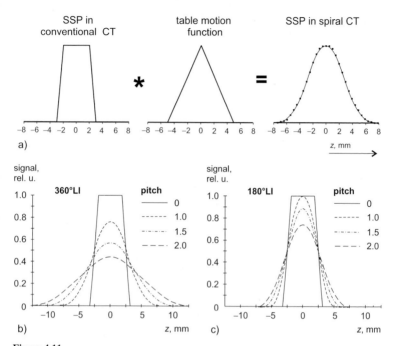

Figure 4.11
Slice sensitivity profiles in spiral CT (5 mm nominal slice width).
a) The SSP in spiral CT results from convolution of the original profile with a triangular motion function.
b), c) Calculated SSPs for 360°LI (**b**) and 180°LI (**c**) as a function of pitch.

The FWTM and SPQI best express the quality of the SSPs. In particular, they also indicate that the original profile already deviates from the ideal shape. For example, sequential CT and a 180°LI reconstruction at pitch = 1 both offer the same nominal slice width of 5.0 mm, but different SPQIs. Both fall below 100%, with the spiral CT SSP deviating more strongly from the ideal. The selected figures of merit should therefore be used not only in spiral CT, but also in sequential CT or other sectional imaging procedures in which the differences in quality of SSPs has also not been adequately evaluated. The slice thickness can be given in general as a value pair, namely the nominal slice thickness, specified by the FWHM, and a figure of merit, such as the SPQI.

4.2.4   Spatial Resolution in the *z*-Direction

As already discussed for the case of sequential CT, the nominal slice thickness is mostly cited as the figure of merit for the resolution in the direction of table advance. While the resolution in fact depends above all on the

Table 4.3
Figures of merit for SSP measurements in sequential CT and in spiral CT, with a nominal slice collimation of 5 mm in each case.

Figure of merit	Sequential CT	Spiral-CT	
		360° LI	180° LI
Pitch = 1			
FWHM, mm	5.0	6.3	5.0
FWTM, mm	6.1	11.1	8.0
FWTA, mm	5.0	8.3	5.9
SPQI, %	93	65	78
Pitch = 2			
FWHM, mm	5.0	10.8	6.5
FWTM, mm	6.1	19.8	11.3
FWTA, mm	5.0	14.1	8.4
SPQI, %	93	42	65

selected slice collimation, it also depends strongly on the scan or reconstruction increment between the individual slice images and the shape of the SSP. These relationships are of fundamental importance and are valid for other slice imaging modalities as well. For spiral CT they have a particular importance, which justifies their detailed treatment in this section.

The broadening of the SSP must be viewed as a disadvantage of spiral CT, while the availability of overlapping images is certainly an essential advantage. The interplay of these factors is decisive. The influence of the slice thickness S and the reconstruction increment RI will be discussed in the next two sections and its fundamental importance explained and illustrated for the example of small lesions.

4.2.4.1 Imaging of lesions

A conventional CT examination yields a fixed number of images, with the distance between two scans usually equal to the slice thickness. In spiral CT, it is possible to freely select the number and the z-positions of the images to be reconstructed within the scan volume. While the broadening of the SSP in spiral CT may negatively affect the contrast and the spatial resolution in a single image (see figure 4.7a), simple considerations show that the availability of images for every position within the scan volume sufficiently compensates for this potential disadvantage.

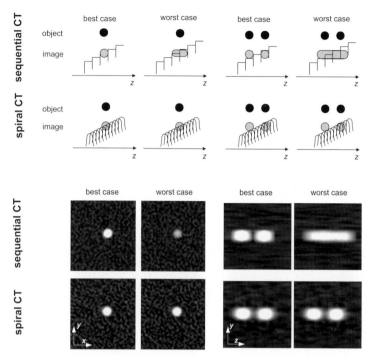

Figure 4.12
Considerations and experiments on contrast and spatial resolution in sequential CT and spiral CT: Spiral CT can always provide the maximum obtainable contrast for a lesion, as follows from basic considerations (top row) and is confirmed by experiments (bottom row) [Kalender, 1994b].

As a thought experiment this will be explained for a situation which occurs often in radiology: searching for a lesion, for example a solitary nodule in the lung. For the sake of simplicity, we will assume a spherical nodule, with a diameter equal to the slice thickness of 5 mm, and that the contrast is 100 % relative to the surrounding material. It is well known that the contrast actually obtained in CT images depends on the position of the nodule in relation to the scanned slice. The maximum contrast is obtained only if the nodule is located at the center of the slice. In practice, however, nodules occur at randomly distributed locations, which are not known. Viewed realistically, then, we find nodules between the best – maximum contrast, with the nodule at the center of the slice – and the worst case – contrast dropping off to 1/2 the maximum value, because the signal is distributed exactly between two slices (figure 4.12 upper left). The examination result will therefore always depend on the fortuitously selected start position of the scan series in relation to the position of the nodule. In spiral CT, on the other hand, one always obtains the maximum possible contrast of a nodule at every position within the scan volume, regardless of the start position for the volume scan, since the images can be reconstructed overlapping with arbitrarily fine reconstruction increments for every arbitrary, and also retrospectively selectable, position (figure 4.12 upper left).

The spatial separation of structures such as neighboring vascular or bony details in the z-direction represents a similar situation. If we continue with the thought experiment above, we now assume two identical spherical objects with a diameter of 5 mm, separated by a distance of 5 mm (figure 4.12 upper right), then the obtainable certainty of separation of the objects in a series of sequential 5 mm slices will again depend on the relative position of the fortuitously selected start position of the scan series in relation to the position of the spherical objects. In the most favorable case the spheres will be perfectly separated, and in the least favorable case the two objects will be imaged as a continuous object, which is distributed with half the contrast of a single sphere over four neighboring slices. In spiral mode, however, the separation of the spheres is assured, independently of the start position for the scan, provided only that the reconstruction increment is chosen to be sufficiently small.

An experimental verification of this thought experiment can be carried out with a phantom which permits us to test the system's capability for detecting tiny, randomly distributed objects, thus for example for spherical objects with arbitrary contrast and diameter positioned at arbitrary locations in three-dimensional space. In the experiment conducted, spherical objects with a contrast of about +260 HU and 5 mm diameter were attached to water-equivalent rods. In this way, the situations depicted above could be realistically simulated. The situations for the best and worst cases postulated at the top of figure 4.12 were easily simulated for individual spheres placed at arbitrary z-positions in a 20 cm water phantom. The contrast, that is the CT value measured at the center of a 5 mm spherical object, varied in the conventional scanning technique for shifted 5 mm slices by a factor of about 2 (best case: 253 HU, worst case: 135 HU). With spiral scans, by comparison, the maximum contrast was always obtained, regardless of the start position. By way of comparison, due to the broadening of the SSP the contrast was 0.89 times the best possible case for sequential CT (reduced to 224 HU). Compared with the worst case for sequential CT, the contrast in spiral CT was superior by a factor of 1.66. The ability of spiral CT to separate two spherical objects arranged along the z-axis also confirmed expectations. Spiral CT therefore demonstrated its superior performance here as well (figure 4.12 lower right).

It goes without saying that the considerations above can be extended in an entirely analogous way to any arbitrary combinations of sphere diameters and slice thicknesses. The advantages of spiral CT derive from the continuous volume scan and are clearly evident whenever making use of the possibility to reconstruct images at arbitrary positions along the z-axis. In clinical practice this is utilized in so far as the radiologist chooses the optimum image, e.g. by means of interactive MPR (see section 6.2), in which the nodule or any other pathological detail is best displayed. The possibility to obtain images with a small reconstruction increment therefore more than compensates for the disadvantage which the smoothed SSP entails in spiral CT.

4.2.4.2   Influence of slice width and reconstruction increment

The predominant influence of the slice thickness on the resolution in the z-direction is largely known; this is because an averaging over all structures located in a slice always takes place. Multiplanar reconstructions on a semi-anthropomorphic test phantom demonstrate this in a simple way (figure 4.13, left column). The geometrically defined European Spine Phantom (ESP) [Kalender, 1995b] used here is especially suited to the assessment of image quality since all geometric parameters, such as the height of 4 mm for the intervertebral space, are exactly known.

The influence of the reconstruction increment RI, i.e. the distance of separation between the positions of neighboring images, is not equally well known but of great importance. The reconstruction of overlapping images brings fundamental advantages with regard to 3D spatial resolution and also diagnostic reliability, in accordance with the experiment shown in figure 4.12. A 50 % overlap, that is a reconstruction increment of half a slice thickness, is a good value for orientation in spiral CT ($RI = S/2$, i.e. two images per slice thickness). An image reconstruction increment equal to the slice thickness ($RI = S$) corresponds to sequential CT and does not utilizes the special advantages of spiral CT. A strongly pronounced overlapping (e.g. $RI = S/3$ or 67 % overlap) is advantageous for high 3D spatial resolution and for excellent MPR and 3D images. This is particularly evident in a direct comparison of reconstructions $RI = 3$ mm and $RI = 1$ mm for $S = 3$ mm (Figure 4.13, center row). In principle, still more strongly overlapping brings further advantages; these considerations and measurements have been extended and quantified [Kalender, 1994b]. In practice, however, the incremental gain in resolution in the z-direction with $RI < S/3$ is too small to justify the effort required.

Therefore I would like to propose a pragmatically oriented 1-2-3 rule. In uncritical cases, one image per slice thickness can be altogether sufficient; this corresponds to sequential CT and accepts a certain loss of resolution and small-detail contrast. Two images per slice thickness should be routinely reconstructed, since this improves diagnostic reliability. Three images per slice thickness are recommended whenever high 3D resolution is demanded. This recommendation applies equally to single-slice and multi-slice spiral CT. The problem of handling the resulting numbers of images and which forms of display are available will be dealt with in chapter 6.

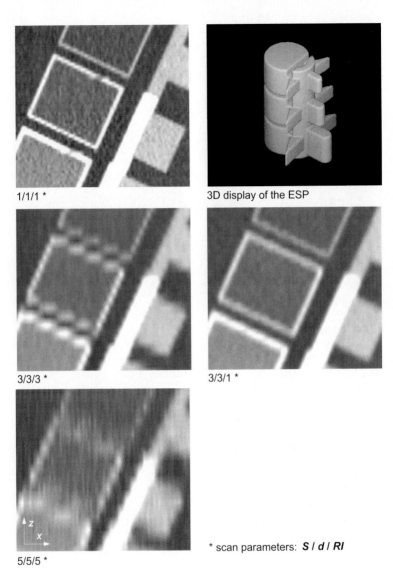

1/1/1 *

3D display of the ESP

3/3/3 *

3/3/1 *

5/5/5 *

* scan parameters: **S / d / RI**

Figure 4.13
Spatial resolution in the z-direction, demonstrated by secondary reconstructions of the European Spine Phantom (upper right). The influence of slice thickness dominates and is evident in the left column for scans with slice thicknesses of 1, 3 and 5 mm, pitch = 1 and $RI = S$. The influence of the reconstruction increment is demonstrated in the second row for scans with $S = 3$ mm reconstructed with $RI = 3$ mm (left) and 1 mm (right), respectively.

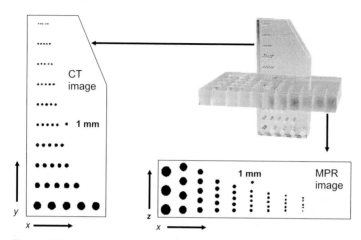

Figure 4.14
Spiral CT can provide isotropic 3D spatial resolution. I.e., resolution is approximately the same in all directions, in the x/y-scan plane as well as in arbitrary multiplanar reformations (scan with $S = 1$ mm, $d = 1$ mm; reconstruction with standard convolution kernel and $RI = 0.4$ mm.)

4.2.4.3   Isotropic 3D spatial resolution

The possibilities for the measurement of the spatial resolution in the slice and perpendicular to the slice were already discussed in section 4.1. In order to acquire both parameters in a single measurement, two high-contrast drilled hole phantoms can be used, for example, one oriented in the x/y-scan plane and the other in the z-direction. The investigations can be repeated for arbitrary settings of the scan and reconstruction parameters. Figure 4.14 shows that spiral CT with suitable parameters enables us to obtain isotropic resolution in the sub-millimeter range to a good approximation, which cannot be obtained in practice with sequential CT. High resolution in the z-direction requires, in addition to thin slices, the reconstruction of several images per slice thickness and the use of a 180° algorithm.

For image reconstruction in spiral CT it is always necessary to define two parameter sets, which are fundamentally independent but which must be matched to each other:

1. the type of z-interpolation, the reconstruction increment and – when z-filtering is used – the effective slice thickness of the images

2. the usual parameters for image reconstruction, such as the convolution kernel, zoom factor and center of the field of view.

The first parameter set influences the quality of the 3D-image stack predominantly in the z-direction, and the second parameter set influences the characteristics of the single images in the x/y-plane. Isotropic spatial resolution is, especially with multi-slice spiral CT, easily achievable even in clinical routine.

4.2.5 Artifacts in Spiral CT

With respect to artifacts in spiral CT, the fundamental considerations discussed at the outset concerning image quality must be taken into account again. The scanner and its physical properties remain unchanged; in most cases artifacts (see section 4.1.5) therefore show the same behavior in sequential CT as in spiral CT. For example, it is to be expected that beam hardening artifacts occur in the same form, and sampling effects within the scan plane should influence the image in the same way.

Before the introduction of spiral CT it had been assumed that moving the patient represented a particularly difficult problem. In practice, however, it was shown that this is not the case. The z-interpolation compensates for the effects of table movement. The effects of possible patient movements on the transverse slice images are not significantly intensified in spiral CT, since the scanner typically works with rotation times of one second or less. For an image obtained through z-interpolation, data are acquired over a maximum time of two seconds, which is still less than the time required in CT for many years for the acquisition of a slice image. The effects of patient movement on multiplanar and 3D-displays of organs and body regions subject to motion are decisively reduced in spiral CT, since these regions are acquired continuously, in a much faster time than was possible with sequential CT. Consequently, patient movement poses no special problem for spiral CT.

Nevertheless, there are effects or artifacts which occur only in spiral CT and, to a certain extent, depend on the type of z-interpolation employed. Because of the broadening of the SSP in spiral CT, it must be expected that partial volume effects are intensified. This represents a potential cause for the deterioration of image quality, such as for the display of bones or for images acquired in the vicinity of the base or the top of the skull, in other words in situations in which the use of thin slices is recommended in sequential CT scans. In spiral CT, such cases also require selecting thin slices, 180° algorithms and pitch values less than 1.5. The broadening of the SSP can influence the contrast and the spatial resolution for small structures in single transverse images. The possibility to select the optimum reconstruction position within the scan volume retrospectively, however, more than compensates for this disadvantage (see section 4.2.4).

Other more subtle effects or artifacts have been observed in spiral CT, for which the z-interpolation and not the broadening of the SSP is evidently responsible. Artifacts in scans of ramp phantom were already mentioned [Polacin, 1994]; there are however no reports in the literature of such artifacts disturbing during clinical examinations. Nonetheless, there is no doubt about the existence of effects, such as hypodense areas in the vicinity of bifurcations in the bronchial tree at higher values of pitch, which can simulate tiny emphysema bullae and can most likely be attributed to inter-polation errors.

More frequently observed are an inhomogeneous distribution of the pixel noise and also of the spatial resolution in the image. As already discussed in section 3.3.3, these effects are scarcely noticeable in a single image, but can be found in maximum intensity projection images in CT angiography (figure 3.5a). Beam hardening has been suggested as a possible cause, al-though other possible error sources such as scattered radiation and pulsat-ing movements have also been proposed. It can safely be assumed that the inhomogeneous distribution of the pixel noise within the field of measure-ment, which varies in a rotating fashion with the z-position, is solely responsible. These effects are seen to grow with increasing distance from the isocenter, but remain relatively modest and can be reduced with the use of suitable z-interpolation algorithms (figure 3.5b).

In summary, we can state that the artifacts which occur in spiral CT are so subtle that they become visible primarily only in 3D and MPR displays. It is entirely clear that they do not create any more frequent or any more significant problems than are already known from sequential CT. This applies equally to both single-slice and multi-slice spiral CT.

4.2.6   Considerations for Multi-slice Spiral CT

For MSCT there are no fundamental changes or deviations as compared to single-slice spiral CT. Those differences which are observed depend on the choice and implementation of the z-interpolation by the particular manu-facturer, for which detailed information is mostly treated as confidential. In spite of this, a few basic statements of general validity can be made.

With the use of a simple linear z-interpolation between the two measured values lying closest to the image position, that is 180°MLI (see section 3.4.1), the noise and sensitivity profile should behave in much the same way as with 180°LI: the σ values are independent of the pitch, and the SSP half-value width increases continuously with the pitch. As explained in sec-tion 3.4.2, however, this approach is hardly ever utilized, since it can lead to image quality problems. Also, there may be peaks in the sensitivity pro-files' FWHM values for pitch values of 0.5 and 1.0 due to the redundant sampling pattern for these choices.

The concept of z-filtering over several of the measured values lying closest to the image position, that is 180°MFI, allows for different implementations (see section 3.4.2). That this could possibly cause pronounced changes in image quality depending on the pitch factor has so far only been postulated [Hu, 1999], but not yet proven. Our experience indicates that this cannot be the case in general. The specific situation for the Siemens Volume Zoom is documen-ted in figure 4.15. SSP quality is essentially constant; only for thin effective slice widths and pitch values >1.75 the FWHM values increase. Noise is also kept constant since the mA value is increased linearly with the pitch value.

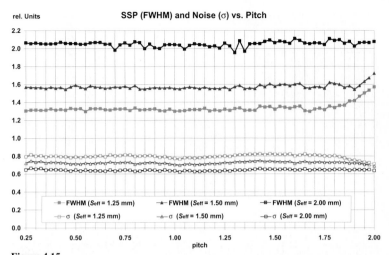

Figure 4.15
The z-resolution, measured as the FWHM of the SSP (upper graphs), and the image noise (lower graphs) show no variation (SOMATOM Volume Zoom) when varying the pitch continuously. Thus, image quality remains independent of the pitch and there is no preferred pitch value in MSCT.

It can be concluded that in MSCT – with adequate z-filtering – there are no preferred values for the pitch factor [Schaller 2000; Fuchs, 2000]. This situation is not only expected physically, but also desirable from the standpoint of clinical routine, since the pitch must be adapted to the examination and not the opposite. This means in general that the SSPs are independent of pitch. Whether the image noise should also be independent of pitch is a question of philosophy. Apparently, the situation for MSCT with z-filtering has changed: in single-slice spiral CT and in MSCT with 180°MLI, always two data points are used for z-interpolation; in MSCT with z-filtering for a given filter width W the number of data points accessed will change when changing the pitch. If the manufacturer compensates for this by a respective change in mA, as is done on the SOMATOM Volume Zoom, noise values independent of the pitch value are provided. This means that image quality and patient dose are largely independent of the pitch value. Of course, when keeping all other scan parameters constant, which has been and will remain the standard in single-slice spiral CT, an increase of the pitch factor leads to a reduction in dose (see section 5.2).

MSCT permits great flexibility in routine applications, since scans with thin slices are nevertheless possible routinely with short volume scan times. By combining slices, low-noise images can be acquired which are almost free of partial volume artifacts and exhibit high contrast resolution (figure 4.16a). Zoom reconstructions of single slices with a high-resolution convolution kernel, on the other hand, yield high spatial resolution (figure 4.16b). Excellent contrast and z-resolution result for a moderate effective

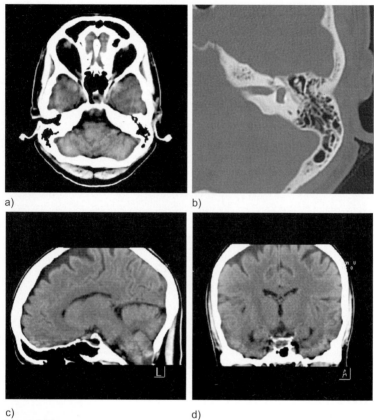

a)   b)

c)   d)
Figure 4.16
Flexibility in MSCT. One spiral scan (4 × 1 mm) can provide distinctly different image
characteristics.
a) z-filtering to calculate 4 mm sections yields high contrast resolution.
b) Selective reconstruction of single 1.25 mm slices yields high spatial resolution.
c, d) MPR images with a 2.5 mm effective slice thickness yields images with high contrast
and z-resolution.

slice thickness of 2.5 mm (figure 4.16c, d). Practically all diagnostic needs
can be satisfied without the need for any additional scans.

4.3 Constancy Tests and Acceptance Testing

CT is a well established procedure in radiology. Requirements for the system characteristics and the type and extent of quality control measurements
should therefore be defined accordingly in national and international standards. It must be stated that this has not yet been done in all points and
that, in particular, spiral CT has not yet been adequately considered.

Table 4.4
Parameters for acceptance testing and constancy testing in CT

Parameter or function	Acceptance testing[1]	Constancy testing[2]
X-ray tube voltage	x	-
CT values	x	x
Homogeneity	x	x
Noise	x	x
Spatial resolution	x	x
Low-contrast resolution	x	-
Slice thickness	x	x
Dose profiles	x	-
Dose on the system axis	x	x
Dose for survey radiographs	x	-
Accuracy of table position	x	x
Gantry tilt	x	-
Light localizers	x	-

[1] Acceptance testing in accordance with DIN 6868, Part 53, December 1990
[2] Constancy testing in accordance with IEC 1223-2-6, April 1994
Note: The presently valid standards make no mention of spiral CT!

The following standards apply in Germany for acceptance testing and constancy testing:

Acceptance testing: DIN 6868, Part 53, valid since December 1990

Constancy testing: IEC 1223-2-6, valid since April 1994

The parameters tested are summarized in table 4.4. In agreement with numerous recommendations and publications, both types of testing cover the essential considerations for sequential CT, while there is no mention whatever of spiral CT.

The reasons for and frequencies of performing test measurements are prescribed. Acceptance testing must be performed at the time of initial installation and whenever substantial modifications are made to the scanning system, such as replacing the x-ray tube. This requirement must be satisfied before beginning or resuming the examination of patients. The values determined must agree with those specified by the manufacturer and then serve as the basis for all further constancy testing. Constancy testing must be performed in monthly intervals. Exceptions to this are the measurement of dose, which is performed semi-annually, and the measurement of spatial resolution, which must be performed quarter-yearly.

For sequential CT, additions or modifications would be desirable in two points:

1. The evaluation of low-contrast measurements is extremely subjective; the different phantoms on the market give widely different results, rendering the testing of acceptance criteria unreliable (see section 4.1.4). A revision of the situation would be desirable.

2. At the international level, dose measurements are still defined differently; acceptance testing requires a measurement free in air on the system axis, whereas constancy testing requires a measurement of the *CTDI* in a phantom. A uniform method of measurement and unequivocal definitions would be desirable (see section 5.2.6).

For spiral CT, standardized procedures are altogether nonexistent. For the characterization of the different implementations in single-slice and multi-slice spiral CT a number of parameters should be acquired, as already discussed above. These include the pixel noise, the homogeneity of the noise, the slice sensitivity profiles and the extended testing of table advance and speed.

In fact a new manufacturer's standard does exist, the IEC standard 60601-2-44 of February 1999 [IEC, 1999]. However, this makes no reference to acceptance and constancy testing in accordance with legal requirements and is not legally binding in regard to this point. Consequently, in the field of CT, particularly with a view to such new technologies as multi-slice spiral CT, there is still work to be done on standards and regulations.

5   Dose

5.1   CT – a High Dose Examination Procedure?

CT is generally associated with high performance in radiological diagnostics, but also with high dose. The classification "high dose examination procedure" is not immediately understandable, as will be shown below. Nevertheless, this has to be viewed in the meantime as an official statement: the Council of the European Union has determined in its "Council Directive 97/43/EURATOM of June 30, 1997 on health protection of individuals against the dangers of ionizing radiation in relation to medical exposure" [European Communities, 1997] in article 9, section (1):

> *"Member states shall ensure that appropriate radiological equipment, practical techniques and ancillary equipment are used in the medical exposure*
>
> *– of children,*
>
> *– as part of a health screening programme,*
>
> *– involving high doses to the patient, such as interventional radiology, computed tomography or radiotherapy.*
>
> *Special attention shall be given to the quality assurance programmes, including quality control measures and patient dose or administered activity assessment, ..."*

CT is placed in the same category here with interventional radiology and with radiotherapy. Also – but this can be viewed favorably – quality assurance and the assessment of patient dose will be required by law in the European Union as of May 13, 2000. What is the justification for these decisions? What are the consequences which will have to follow?

Contrary to the general expectations that, with the advent of magnetic resonance imaging and its widespread use the usefulness of x-ray computed tomography would quickly decline, CT continues to gain in its importance. The introduction of spiral CT and the technical improvements which this brought have led to a veritable renaissance of CT. The range of CT applications has been extended, for example through CT angiography and through multiphase contrast studies. The recent introduction of multi-row detectors has once again drastically increased the performance capability and further simplified CT examinations. Thus, there is every reason to expect a continued increase in the number of CT examinations.

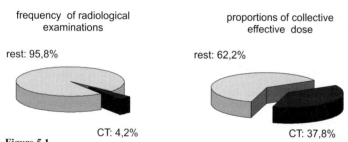

frequency of radiological
examinations

proportions of collective
effective dose

rest: 95,8%

rest: 62,2%

CT: 4,2%

CT: 37,8%

Figure 5.1
Although CT examinations make up only a relatively small part of the total number of x-ray examinations, CT contributes a high proportion of the collective effective dose. The figures shown refer to Germany for the year 1994 [BMU, 1996], but can be taken as largely representative for most western countries.

The relative contribution of CT to the dose per capita arising from medical examinations will of course increase proportionately. Although CT examinations make up only three to five percent of all radiological examinations, their contribution to the total dose in the western world amounts to about 35 to 45 percent [BMU, 1996; Kaul, 1997; Royal Coll. Radiologists, 1998] (figure 5.1). For this reason, CT is subject to the particular scrutiny of radiation protection measures; there are demands to limit or reduce the dose levels arising in the use of CT [Bauer, 1998; European Commission's Study Group, 1998]. This development also constitutes the background for the new EU directive referred to above in regard to the protection of persons against the dangers of ionizing radiation during exposure for medical purposes. Along with the classification of CT as a "medical exposure ... involving high doses to the patient", the assessment of patient dose and the establishment of and adherence to binding reference dose values has been defined. The lawmakers in the countries of the European Union must create the corresponding regulations by May 13, 2000!

In keeping with the fundamental and current importance of the subject of dose in CT, this chapter is devoted to a detailed discussion of the dose-relevant aspects of CT. In particular, information will be made available which can be of help for conducting the necessary discussions with professional colleagues, as well as with patients and the public in general.

5.2   Technical Parameters for Dose Measurement

The parameters for the physical measurements of dose in CT were established long ago. These are

- the dose distribution in the scan plane, $D(x,y)$,

- the dose distribution normal to the scan plane, the dose profile $D(z)$,

- and the dose distribution in space, the stray radiation $D(x,y,z)$.

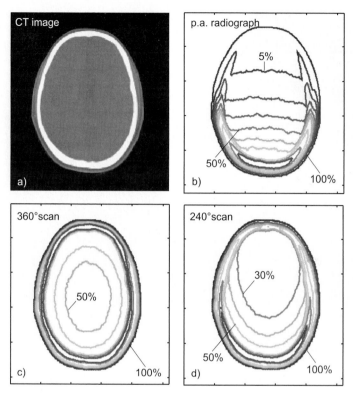

Figure 5.2
Dose distributions in the cranial slice shown **(a)** calculated by Monte Carlo methods for conventional x-ray **(b)**, for a CT scan over 360° **(c)** and for a 240° partial scan **(d)**.

The first two parameters are directly concerned with the patient, while the third is primarily of interest for the assessment of exposure to the examiner and for radiation protection considerations. These parameters, defined and determined for sequential CT, also permit a complete description of the situation for spiral CT and multi-slice spiral CT when taking account of a few special aspects. Some detail questions, for example whether dose should be specified in air, in water, in tissue or even in plexiglas, which have not been finally answered yet, will be discussed in section 5.2.6.

5.2.1   Sequential Single-slice Scans

For conventional x-ray images, the dose falls off from the point of entry to the point of exit according to the behavior of the primary intensity, but with scattered radiation components superimposed, i.e. exponentially to a good approximation (figure 5.2a, b). With CT, however, the corresponding con-

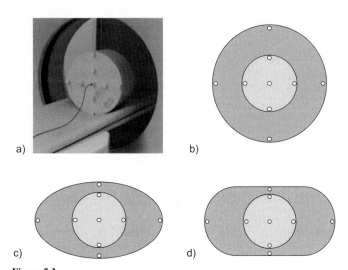

Figure 5.3
The dose distribution in the acquired slice is determined using CTDI phantoms.
a, b) Standard phantoms with 16 and 32 cm diameters.
c, d) Phantoms made of water-equivalent plastic with cross-sections more closely approximating anthropomorphic conditions, thus enabling a more realistic estimate of dose.

tributions from all projections acquired over the 360° measurement are summed; the resulting dose distribution in the slice examined, $D(x,y)$, is consequently relatively homogeneous (figure 5.2c). Here as well, the dose at the points of entry, that is over the entire outer surface, is higher than in the center. However, the greatest variations occurring are by a factor of 2 to 5 and not by orders of magnitude. Only for partial scans over a limited angular range does a more pronounced asymmetry of the distribution result (figure 5.2d).

Just as for CT values and for noise, dose must also be measured at different positions in the phantom and for different-sized phantoms. For this purpose, the CTDI phantom has become the established standard (*CTDI* – Computed Tomography Dose Index) [Shope, 1981]. It is specified with diameters of 16 cm and 32 cm in order to approximate the attenuation conditions for head and body examinations and has an axial extent of at least 14 cm (figure 5.3a, b). CTDI phantoms are made of plexiglas or water-equivalent plastic. In addition to a central bore, four peripheral bores at a depth of 10 mm are provided. In addition to the determination of the dose distribution in the slice at the selected points of measurement, performed with pencil ionization chambers, it is also possible to measure the dose profile in the z-direction at these positions.

The dose profile, similar to the sensitivity profile, is determined largely by the focus size, the scanner geometry and especially by the primary collimation (figure 2.6). The sensitivity profile is somewhat narrower than the dose profile, especially when a collimator is employed on the detector side, which of course affects only the sensitivity profile and not the dose profile. Furthermore, as a result of scattered radiation the dose profiles show long-range tails. For physical reasons, this effect is unavoidable and depends on the size of the object and on the slice thickness. Just as in conventional radiography, this leads to the exposure of organs outside the region examined. In order to assess these influences, it is necessary to measure the total dose profile $D(z)$ and not only the dose within the slice acquired.

The measurement of dose profiles is performed mostly at the center only, either free in air with x-ray film or in CTDI phantoms with thermoluminescence dosimeters (TLD). The measurement with x-ray film is performed fast and easily, but permits only a qualitative check of the collimator widths and is used primarily for constancy checking. A reliable quantification is not possible with film. On the other hand, TLD measurements require considerable effort and, because of the differences in the spectral components in the primary radiation and scattered radiation fields, are also problematic. Simpler procedures, such as with electronic sensors, are in the development stage, but are not yet available on a wide basis.

Figure 5.4 shows several dose profiles measured with TLD. The left column shows measurements free in air, with which – as for constancy checking with film – the collimation can be checked. The measurements in the phantom with diameters of 16 cm and 32 cm show that there is a considerable contribution to the dose outside of the directly exposed slice as a result of scattered radiation, which, as has to be expected, increases with slice thickness and object diameter.

Because of the scattered radiation contributions and because the full width at half maximum of the dose profile is often slightly greater than that of the sensitivity profile, for a series of contiguous slices an excess dose results compared with the dose expected from a single slice (figure 5.5). This means, as a rule, that the maximum value of the dose profile for a slice is not an indication of the peak dose values which can be expected for the entire examination. In order to estimate the dose resulting from a multiple slice or volume examination, the "Multiple Slice Average Dose" (MSAD) was proposed, which is determined for the number of slices and the scan increment I chosen for the particular examination:

$$MSAD = \frac{1}{I} \cdot \int_{-\infty}^{+\infty} D(z)dz. \tag{5.1}$$

The underlying idea of the MSAD has become a standard in the form of the CT dose index. The first definition was advanced by the Food and Drug Administration in the USA (FDA) and has been anchored in USA's legislation in the following form [Shope, 1981]:

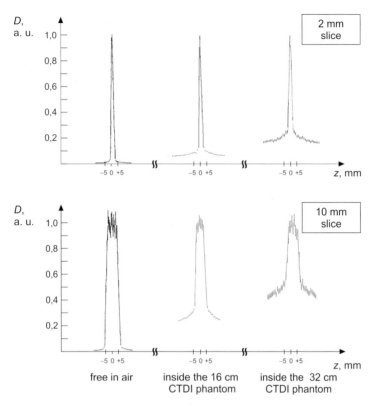

Figure 5.4
Dose profiles for different slice thicknesses, measured with thermoluminescence dosimeters at the center of rotation and in the center of the phantom. As expected, the scattered radiation contributions increase with slice thickness and phantom diameter.

$$CTDI_{FDA} = \frac{1}{S} \cdot \int_{-7S}^{+7S} D(z)dz. \tag{5.2}$$

With the *CTDI*, the dose contributions outside of the directly exposed slice are also taken into account. Therefore again, as a rule, the *CTDI* value is greater than the peak value of the dose profile (figure 5.5). While the basic idea of the *CTDI* is generally accepted, the FDA definition was only necessarily accepted by the manufacturers aiming for the USA market and entails both practical and fundamental problems. Practical problems in measuring result from the variable integration limits, which depend on the particular slice thickness S, since ionisation chambers are not available in arbitrary lengths of $14 \cdot S$. Typically, the measurements are made with ionization chambers 10 cm in length. This makes a correction to the measured values necessary, which requires a knowledge of the entire dose profile. This effort is frequently unacceptably high, for example within the scope of constancy checking.

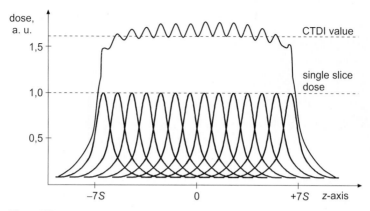

Figure 5.5
For the acquisition of several neighboring slices, a dose excess results compared with the dose expected from any single slice, as shown qualitatively in the sketch.

The essential problem in the definition of the $CTDI_{FDA}$ arises due to the fact that, because of the variable integration limits, defined in relation to the nominal slice thickness, for thin slices a smaller scatter volume is included than for thick slices. Thus, for thin slices, this leads to an incorrect underestimation. This problem is well known. Especially at the European level and in standards committees new proposals have been developed, which provide for a fixed integration length of 100 mm [European Commission's Study Group, 1998]:

$$_nCTDI_{100,x} = \frac{1}{S} \cdot \int_{-50\,mm}^{+50\,mm} D(z)dz. \tag{5.3}$$

the subscript n indicates that the *CTDI* value is normalized with respect to a standard mAs product, usually per 100 mAs. The subscript 100 indicates the integration length of 100 mm. The subscript x indicates whether the measured values are given for air (x = air) or for a phantom at the center (x = c), on the periphery (x = p) or weighted (x = w).

The measurement of the dose free in air, the so-called air kerma value, still required in the Federal Republic of Germany for acceptance testing in CT, thus corresponds to the definition

$$_nCTDI_{100,\,air} = \frac{1}{S} \cdot \int_{-50\,mm}^{+50\,mm} D(z)dz. \tag{5.4}$$

However, the measurement in the phantom is to be preferred, since this takes better account of the influences of prefiltration and shaped filters.

A weighted sum of the peripheral and central CTDI values has also been proposed [European Commission's Study Group, 1998]:

$$_{n}CTDI_{100,w} = 1/3 \cdot {_{n}CTDI_{100,c}} + 2/3 \cdot {_{n}CTDI_{100,p}}. \tag{5.5}$$

Typical CTDI values are listed in Table 5.1 for different slice thicknesses and CTDI phantoms. The values decrease slightly with slice thickness, since the scatter volume then becomes smaller. For very thin slices, the values again increase. This can be attributed to the slight broadening of the dose profile relative to the sensitivity profile which results in this case.

An evaluation of the dose profile can also be made through a comparison of the half-value widths for the sensitivity profile and the dose profile. The geometrical efficiency of the system in the z-direction can be given by

$$\varepsilon_g = \frac{HWB_{SSP}}{HWB_{DP}} \cdot 100\,\%. \tag{5.6}$$

Ideally, the values are close to 100%; such values can be attained for wide slices. Lower values result from using near-detector collimation. Values of less than 70% must be viewed critically; the user should be informed of such values and made aware of them [IEC, 1999].

Table 5.1
Normalized CTDI values and air kerma values for different slice thicknesses, measured centrally and peripherally in 16 cm and 32 cm plexiglas CTDI phantoms at 120 kVp on a SOMATOM PLUS 4.

Slice thickness [mm]	$_{n}CTDI_{100,c}$ [mGy/100mAs]	$_{n}CTDI_{100,p}$ [mGy/100mAs]	$_{n}CTDI_{w}$ [mGy/100mAs]	Air kerma [mGy/100mAs]
16 cm CDTI phantom				
1	12.1	13.7	13.2	16.9
2	10.5	11.4	11.1	14.0
3	10.7	11.7	11.3	14.5
5	11.2	12.3	11.9	15.2
8	11.3	12.2	11.9	15.3
10	11.4	12.3	12.0	15.5
32 cm CDTI phantom				
1	4.4	9.1	7.5	16.9
3	3.8	7.9	6.5	14.5
10	4.1	8.3	6.9	15.5

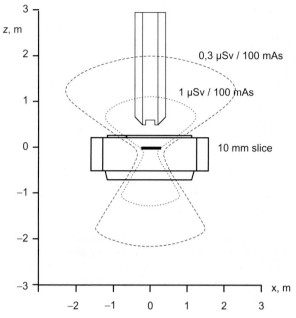

Figure 5.6
Typical distribution of the stray radiation rate. Shown are the isodose lines for every 100 mAs for a SOMATOM PLUS 4 at 10 mm collimation. The exposure resulting from scattered radiation in the examination room is lowest at the side of the gantry.

5.2.2   Volume Scans

The normalized CTDI value characterizes the particular CT scanner. It can also be used, however, to obtain a first estimate of the dose characterizing a complete examination. For this purpose, the dose length product (DLP) has been proposed [European Commission's Study Group, 1998]:

$$DLP = \sum_{i} C_i \cdot {}_nCTDI_{100,\,w,i} \cdot N_i \cdot S_i. \tag{5.7}$$

The summation symbol means that the contributions of all scanning sequences i of an examination, thus for example the plain scan and the contrast scan, must be considered. C_i indicates the individual mAs value, N_i the number of sequential scans or spiral rotations, respectively, and S_i the individual slice thickness. The definition of the dose length product in the form above is therefore suitable for use with the sequential scanning of an entire volume with single scans, as well as for spiral CT. This does not permit any direct assessment of the patient dose, however, since it does not take the specific anatomical regions scanned into account.

5.2.3   Stray Radiation

The dose distribution in the vicinity of the scanner, the so-called stray radiation, is the result of scattered radiation originating from the patient or object scanned and possibly also of leakage radiation. The determination of stray radiation levels is important for radiation protection considerations and serves to estimate the level of exposure of the examining personnel, in case they must remain with the patient during the examination. In the control room and in adjoining rooms and areas, the stray radiation is also determined as part of acceptance testing in order to determine whether the intended operation will conform with all legal limit values for radiation protection.

Whenever examination personnel must be present in the examination room as part of an interventional procedure, for the administration of contrast medium or caring for the patient, the stray radiation distribution is the best indicator for the radiation level to which the personnel is potentially exposed (figure 5.6). The dose rate values are in particular very low when the person remains largely in the "shadow" of the gantry. The dose can be estimated using the mAs product. For a position at a point with stray radiation rate of 0.5 μSv/100 mAs, for example, for 40 scans, each with 250 mAs, a stray radiation value of 50 μSv results. This value applies, for example, for the lens of the eye, which is usually unprotected, whereas the greatest part of the body's surface is protected by the lead apron.

5.2.4   Special Considerations for Spiral CT Scans

From the physical and technical point of view, for spiral CT there are no new or unexpected aspects with regard to dose. To date, no special methods of measurement or parameters have been defined for spiral CT, and there does not appear to be any particular requirement for these. There are of course no dose profiles such as for single slice scans. For central points, the distribution in the z-direction is absolutely smooth and does not show the peaks (contiguous scanning of slices with increments equal to the nominal slice width – compare figure 5.5) or valleys (scanning of representative slices in greater intervals) that occur with sequential scanning, since scanning takes place continuously in spiral CT. Peripherally, spiral scanning leads to a modulation of the dose distribution, which can be easily demonstrated, for example, with the use of x-ray film. This phenomenon is in any case of no special relevance.

Along with the positive aspects which spiral CT offers in regard to patient dose (see section 5.3.2), one particular, but somewhat less important, aspect deserves to be mentioned. With spiral CT, each measured value is in fact used for the image reconstruction. Nevertheless, at the start and the end of the spiral, these contributions are weighted less. Here, a disadvantage could result compared with sequential CT. The situation is illustrated in figure 5.7 for single-slice spiral CT.

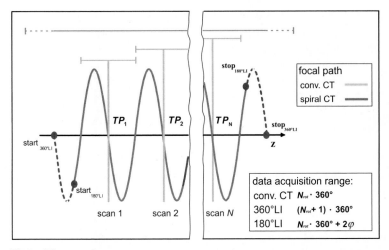

Figure 5.7
Comparison of the scanning regions required for sequential CT and spiral CT. For the usual examination lengths, no significant difference results with regard to the patient dose.

Under the assumption that an organ or section of the body with an extent of N_{rot} slice thicknesses is to be scanned, in sequential CT this requires N_{rot} scans, each over 360° performed at the table positions TP_1 to TP_N. Spiral CT, on the other hand, requires an extended scanning region for each image: for image reconstruction with 360°LI z-interpolation, a data range of 2 · 360° must be available; data must therefore have already been acquired over 360° when TP_1 is reached. Put another way, with sequential CT, at TP_1 data are being acquired over 360°, whereas with spiral CT data are acquired up to TP_1 over 360°. A difference then results when, after reaching TP_N, another 360° of data acquisition are still required for 360°LI. Thus in spiral CT, in the most unfavorable case one additional rotation is required. This must be taken into account for short scanning segments. For a 180°LI reconstruction, the difference reduces to an additional acquisition path of twice the fan angle φ. This can be regarded as negligible and, through modification of the z-interpolation for these end regions, can be completely reduced to zero (e.g. with 180°IX, see table. 3.2). For 180°LI, the most commonly used procedure, for an unusually short spiral scan of only 10 revolutions and a fan angle φ of about 50° there would only be a difference of 2.5 % in the dose, and for normal scans of 25 revolutions or more a difference of less than 1 % as compared to sequential scanning. The dose length product is the appropriate value for a comparison of scan protocols. Along with the different use made of the spiral end segments, the pitch factor also is implicitly taken into account through the number of rotations.

5.2.5   Special Considerations for Multi-slice Spiral CT Scans

There are no fundamental differences between multi-slice spiral CT and single-slice spiral CT in regard to dose. Nevertheless, there are a few points worth mentioning and one important technical difference. As for the definition of the pitch factor, it is necessary to modify the definition of the CTDI value also through taking account of the number M of simultaneously acquired slices:

$$_nCTDI_{100,\,air} = \frac{1}{M \cdot S} \int_{-50\,mm}^{+50\,mm} D(z)dz. \tag{5.8}$$

Here it should be pointed out that equ (5.8) corresponds to the original definition [Rothenberg, 1995], which because of the frequent use of "multi-slice systems" in the early days ($M = 2$, see table 2.4) had to consider the number M. The normalization to $M \cdot S$ is necessary and meaningful because otherwise CTDI values would result which would typically lie above the values commonly known by a factor of M. A comparison between one, two and four row detector systems would otherwise be rendered difficult. In this way, the same arguments apply as for the definition of the pitch factor (compare section 3.2).

The question discussed in section 5.2.4 for single-slice spiral CT of to what extent the exposed examination volumes are greater than the volumes shown in the images is of higher importance in multi-slice spiral CT. The answer is once again dependent on the implementation of the particular manufacturer, for which details are generally not given. Again, it is recommended that the dose length product be used for the purpose of comparisons, since this takes the exposed volumes fully into account. The definition in equ. (5.7) must be extended, however, to include the number of simultaneously acquired slices M_i in each examination, which can also be varied from one examination to another:

$$DLP = \sum_i {}_nCTDI_{100,\,w,i} \cdot N_i \cdot M_i \cdot S_i \cdot C_i. \tag{5.9}$$

The scattered radiation components, and thus the stray radiation, increase for systems with M slices acquired simultaneously and otherwise unchanged exposure parameters by a factor of about M. This is of little relevance, however, since the examination time and the entire mAs product are reduced correspondingly. Consequently, there is no significant difference compared with sequential CT or single-slice spiral CT.

There is a technical problem associated with MSCT in respect to dose, however. To ensure proper normalization of all measured intensity values it is desirable that all detector rows are offered the same primary intensity value I_0. This implies that penumbra regions of the fan beam which are of no or little concern in single-slice CT should be avoided in MCT. This situation is sketched in an exaggerated fashion in figure 5.8. While penumbral radiation intensities are fully utilized in single-slice acquisition, they

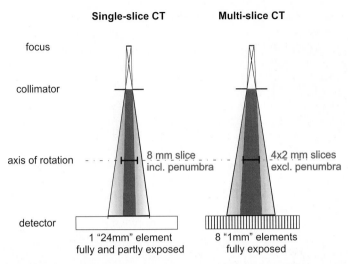

Figure 5.8
While radiation intensity in the penumbral region is fully utilized in single-slice acquisition it is generally excluded in MCT implying a loss in geometric efficiency and a relative increase in CTDI values.

are to be excluded in practical MCT implementations to exclude errors in attenuation measurements. This implies a reduction of geometric efficiency (equ. 5.6) and a corresponding increase in CTDI values. Typical increases of 10 % to 30 % have to be expected depending on the design and the slice width used.

Problems in this respect and significantly higher increases have been reported for one type of MSCT scanner; McCollough et al. measured increases in *CTDI* by more than 100 % for the 4 · 1.25 mm slices [McCollough, 1999]. The manufacturer has meanwhile partly cured the "infant disease". Since real systems are inevitably susceptible to thermal, mechanical or other disturbances, manufacturers try to build in a safety margin by keeping the dose profile wider. Proper control of all system parameters, in particular of the focus position, is the alternative. It will remain a particular challenge for MSCT designers to limit dose increases due to lacking usage of penumbral radiation. The effect's relative importance will decrease with increasing values of $M · S$, i.e. it will be of less significance when wider arrays become available, since the relative proportion of the penumbral region decreases. It will necessarily remain significant for submillimeter slices and small M, e.g. for special collimations such as 2 · 0.5 mm, which should therefore be reserved for high-resolution high-contrast imaging.

5.2.6 Regulations for Dose Measurement

It must be said in general that the applicable regulations so far do not offer uniform procedures for the measurement of dose. In the Federal Republic of Germany, for example, for the constancy check and the acceptance test with CT, the free-in-air measurement of dose, corresponding to equ. 5.4, is still required. The FDA, on the other hand, requires the measurement of the CTDI value in plexiglas phantoms and its specification as a plexiglas energy dose. The IEC requires the measurement of the *CTDI* in plexiglas and its specification as an air energy dose. It would of course be desirable to measure the CTDI value in water and specify this as a water energy dose, since this would most closely resemble the values in human tissue and is also common in other areas of radiology. Water-equivalent phantoms (figure 5.2) are available in the meantime at no additional cost, but so far have not been considered. It remains an open question when there will be a harmonization of standards within Europe or worldwide.

5.3 Patient Dose in CT

Whereas technical dose information is required by law and generally available, information on the patient dose arising for any arbitrary examination has so far been difficult to obtain. The patient dose depends on a number of parameters. In addition to the technical characteristics of the system and the selected examination parameters, it also depends on the size of the patient and the anatomical region selected. This section deals with the dependence of the dose on the selection of the examination parameters and the scanning mode and gives information on the level of the patient dose for different examination types. The possibilities for reducing the dose and efforts towards optimization of procedures will be dealt with in the next section.

5.3.1 Influence of Scanning Parameters on the Patient Dose

Dose depends strongly on the selected x-ray spectrum, that is on the tube voltage and the radiation filtration. It is generally true that, for a given level of image quality, in particular for the same noise level, the patient dose is less with a scanner having a higher effective energy, which results from higher kVp settings or a higher degree of radiation filtration. This behavior is similar to that in conventional radiography; however, the influence on contrast is less critical for CT. It has to be acknowledged that the optimal spectrum for different CT applications has not yet been generally determined.

There is a simple relationship between dose, tube current (mA) and examination time (s): dose is a linear function of the tube current-time product (mAs). A reduction of the mAs value, for example by a factor of two,

Table 5.2 Influences on the patient dose

Parameter	Influence on the patient dose
High tube voltage	Higher kVp values are advantageous (assuming the same image noise level)
Filtration	Higher degree of filtration is advantageous
Tube current	Linear increase in dose with mA value
Scanning time	Linear increase in dose with scanning time
Slice thickness S	Approximately linear increase in dose with S (valid only for single slices!)
Scan volume V	Approximately linear increase in dose with V

reduces the dose at the same rate, but of course also causes an increase in the noise level by a factor of $\sqrt{2}$ (see section 4.2.2). Since in many cases the examination region is defined and all other parameters are held constant, the mAs product is frequently used to estimate the dose. This is possibly meaningful for the relative comparison of examination protocols on the same scanner. As a comparison between different scanners, however, it is misleading and fundamentally incorrect to compare the mAs products in order to arrive at an estimate of the dose. A high degree of prefiltration, which is altogether meaningful for a low patient dose, requires a high mAs product. A manufacturer who is conscious of the patient dose and chooses to use a high degree of filtration in spite of the greater loading of the x-ray components which this entails will be penalized unjustifiably if only the mAs values are compared with one another.

A simple relationship also exists between the exposed volume and the patient dose: the integral dose, given for example as the dose length product, varies essentially linearly with the size of the examination region. Strict linearity no longer applies when such dose values as organ dose or effective dose are determined, because the human body is built up inhomogeneously, and extending the scanning region can acquire information from different organ regions. The important rule of thumb, that the total dose depends linearly on the size of the volume examined, remains unaffected in essence. Therefore, the examination volume should be kept as small as possible.

Of course it is also true by analogy that, when scanning only a single slice or only a few representative slices at greater intervals, the dose increases with the slice thickness. Since in most cases, however, a complete volume is examined the choice of slice thickness has no primary influence. Indirectly, there may be an effect, for example when selecting a higher mAs value with thin slices or if an increased CTDI value is associated with thin slices (see table 5.1). The dependences described are briefly summarized in table 5.2. They apply in equal measure for sequential CT and spiral CT.

Table 5.3
Advantages and disadvantages of spiral CT in regard to dose compared with sequential CT.

Influence	Assumption	Dose in spiral CT
Use of data in first and last segments	>25 rotations, 180°LI	Increased by <1 %
Table feed per revolution ≥ slice thickness	1.0 ≤ pitch factor ≤ 2.0	Reduced by 0–50 %
Overlapping image reconstruction for MPR and 3D displays	33 % or 50 % overlapping	Reduced by 33 % or 50 %, respectively
Changing noise level through z-interpolation	360°LI or 180°LI	Reduced or increased, respectively, by 33 %
Changing noise level through z-interpolation	Adaptive filtering (see section 5.4.2)	Significant reduction for large objects
Use of tube current modulation	Anatomy-dependent and in real-time (see section 5.4.2)	Reduced by 15–60 %

5.3.2 Influence of Spiral CT on Patient Dose

The introduction of volume scanning with spiral CT can be judged positively in every respect. From the standpoint of dose, however, certain reservations have been reported. The simple thought was frequently expressed in the beginning that the patient dose is higher when an entire volume is exposed to radiation instead of single slices. In point of fact, however, sequential CT and spiral CT differ only very little. This is to be expected for the same reasons advanced with respect to the considerations for image quality. With both methods, the dose increases with tube current and tube voltage, scan time and volume examined. The same conversion factors apply for both scanning principles for the conversion of the mAs product to CTDI value and dose. Above all, for comparison purposes it is a necessary and justifiable assumption that the same anatomical region is always examined, regardless of whether this is by means of a spiral scan or a number of single slice scans. For an examination requiring only a few representative slice scans, there is a priori no indication for a spiral examination. All this means that, in general, there is no reason to expect an increase of patient dose for the examination of complete organs or anatomical regions with spiral CT.

On the other hand, practical considerations lead to considerable differences between the two scanning modes and to a positive effect in the sense of a reduction in dose with spiral CT.

- Overlapping scans, which were often selected for good multiplanar or 3D displays and led to corresponding increases in dose, are no longer a necessity because overlapping images are available in spiral CT with no additional exposure.

- Repeat scans, which were frequently required if the patient moved significantly or breathed between single scans, have been practically eliminated by spiral CT.

- The technically available mA values are generally somewhat lower with spiral CT than with sequential CT in order to prevent overheating of the tube over longer scan times (see figure 2.5).

- The selection of pitch factors greater than 1 enables not only scanning a volume in a shorter time, but also results in a reduction in dose corresponding to the pitch factor.

In total, therefore, spiral CT offers the possibility for an effective and efficient dose reduction compatible with routine operation. The most important contribution follows from the selective choice of pitch factors greater than 1; typically these lie in the range 1.2 to 1.6 for standard applications and up to 2.0 in CT angiography or orthopedic examinations. For the contiguous acquisition of volumes, in agreement with equ. (5.7) and (5.9), dose in spiral CT is reduced according to

$$D_{\text{spiral CT}} = D_{\text{conv CT}} / p \ . \tag{5.10}$$

Principally, it must also be considered that, for otherwise identical scanning parameters, the noise level in spiral CT depends on the z-interpolation algorithm (see section 4.2.2). The most commonly used 180°LI algorithm is associated with an increase of about 15 % in noise level. Compensating for this would require an increase of about 33 % in dose. Alternatively, it is also possible to obtain a reduction in noise with the use of other algorithms, such as 360°LI, at the cost of a loss of z-axis resolution. Recent multidimensional adaptively filtering algorithms [Kachelrieß, 1999] and the possibilities discussed in section 3.4.2 for multi-slice spiral CT, however, offer effective alternatives, so that in all there are decisive advantages for spiral CT.

5.3.3   Estimation of Organ Dose Values and Effective Dose

The physical quantities determined by dose-related measurements with phantoms do not permit a simple conversion to patient dose values. The geometry and material of the phantoms can hardly be described as anthropomorphic, and organs are not taken into account. An estimate of the patient dose for CT examinations will nevertheless be required by law in the future, as discussed in section 5.1. This information should in any case be available to the medical staff and to the patient independently of any legal requirements.

Numerous investigations of patient dose can be found in the literature, all of these averaged over a large number of patients as well as different examination conditions and CT scanners. Typical values are given in table 5.4 for a few examinations to provide orientation on the orders of magnitude

Table 5.4
Dose values for a few typical CT examinations. Contiguous single slices or spiral CT with a pitch = 1 are assumed. For a pitch > 1 the dose decreases by a factor of approximately $1/p$.

Anatomical regions	Head	Chest	Abdomen	Pelvis
Scan range, cm	15	31	24	15
Slice thickness, mm	5	5	5	5
Tube current × rotation time, mAs	200	150	250	250
Voltage, kVp	120	140	120	120
Air kerma, mGy/100mAs	13.5	18.4	13.5	13.5
Critical organ	Eye lens	Lung	Liver	Bladder
Organ dose, mSv	22.2	22.1	21.7	19.1
Effective dose, mSv	0.9	6.4	6.8	3.9
Years of natural background radiation at 3 mSv/y.	0.3	2.1	2.3	1.3

to be expected [Kalender, 1999a]. In addition to the organ dose for directly exposed critical organs, the effective dose is also listed, which expresses the sum value over all organs weighted by their radiation sensitivities, according to internationally valid recommendations [ICRP, 1990].

In order to be able to make more precise, examination-specific estimates, calculations have been performed with the Monte Carlo method for 'standard man' by several groups and the results summarized in tables [Shrimpton, 1991; Zankl, 1991]. To present these difficult to read and difficult to interpret tables in a simpler and more useful form, a PC-based program was written which permits the definition of any arbitrary scanning regions and examination parameters and the calculation of the dose values for all organs of interest, as well as the effective dose [Kalender, 1999a]. Calculations for the example of a CT examination of the lung are shown in figure 5.9. A demonstration version of the respective program is included on the CD-ROM for the interested reader to explore the influence of different parameter settings. It has meanwhile been expanded to allow for patient-specific dose calculations based on the actual CT parameter settings and the given CT images (see figure 5.12 below, for example).

An important result is the confirmation that CT examinations can be performed with typical values of the effective dose between 1.0 and 10 mSv. Peak dose values and organ dose values in the directly examined region lie well below 100 mSv and usually below 1 mSv in regions further away. It is

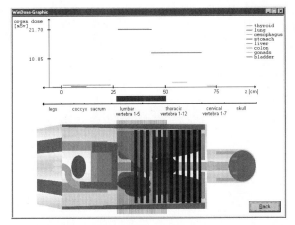

Figure 5.9
The calculation of organ dose values and effective dose is possible without problems for
any arbitrary CT scanning protocol [Kalender, 1999a]. The results can be displayed in
graphical and tabular form. You may explore the program in a reduced version on the
enclosed CD-ROM.

important to note that the values for the effective dose are of the order of
magnitude of natural background radiation. In Germany this is officially
determined at 2.4 mSv per year with a range from 1 to 10 mSv observed for
different regions [BMU, 1996], for the USA the mean value is 3.0 mSv.
Therefore, effective doses in CT can be quoted at typically between 0.2 and 5
times the natural background radiation per year for a single examination. The
dose of course increases for multiple examinations according to equ. (5.8).
This must be given special consideration, for example, with dynamic CT (see
section 2.3.4) or interventional CT (see section 2.3.5). The Monte Carlo calculations referred to above can easily take this into account and determine
dose values for the individual patient on the basis of the CT images.

5.4   Possibilities for Reducing the Dose

Efforts and measures to reduce dose can be initiated

- by the examiner by critically considering the indication and the choice
  of scanning protocols and parameters for any CT examination and

- by the manufacturer during the development of dose-efficient systems,
  together with special technical measures and methods.

The most important points are summarized in table 5.5. Here, it should be
clear that the manufacturer can and should influence the examination protocols, and the user can and should influence the technical measures.

Table 5.5   Possibilities for dose reduction with CT

Measures for the examiner	Measures for the manufacturer
Checking the indication and limiting the scanned volume	Increasing the prefiltration of the radiation spectrum
Adapting the scanning parameters to the patient cross-section	Attenuation-dependent tube current modulation
Pronounced reduction of mAs values for children	Low-dose scanning protocols for children and special indications
Use of spiral CT with pitch factors >1 and calculation of overlapping images instead of acquiring overlapping single scans	Automatic exposure control for sequential CT and spiral CT
Adequate selection of image reconstruction parameters	Noise-reducing image reconstruction procedures
Use of z-filtering with multi-slice CT systems	Further development of algorithms for z-filtering and adaptive filtering

5.4.1   Influence by the Examiner

Even if it appears trivial, it always remains important to emphasize that a great potential for dose reduction is given by scrutinizing the requests for CT examinations with respect to their necessity. The often quoted high values for cumulative dose (figure 5.1) could certainly be reduced somewhat here. It is also important to repeatedly emphasize that, to a first approximation, patient dose is directly proportional to the size of the region examined. Thus, along with the indication, it should also be checked whether it is possible to reduce the volume. Finally, it is hardly necessary to mention that every examination should be performed with the optimum dose, i.e. with the minimum dose necessary to ensure the required image quality. Dose minimization without regard to image quality can lead to image results which are not suitable to diagnosis and should therefore be avoided just as carefully as an unnecessarily high dose.

An absolutely essential measure for the selection of the optimum dose lies in the adaptation of the scanning parameters to the diameter of the patient, as is done in conventional radiology. This is especially true for examinations of children, since considerably lower mAs values and thus effective dose values below 1 mSv should be applied here. The selection of adequate reconstruction parameters, in particular for noise reduction, is important whenever low-contrast presentations are of primary concern.

The specific possibilities which spiral CT offers for the reduction of dose were discussed in the previous section. The most effective measure for dose reduction is given by choosing a pitch factor of greater than 1. The specific use of the new possibilities which multi-slice CT systems offer can

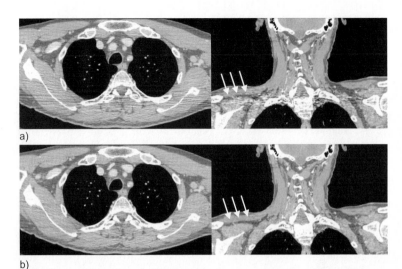

a)

b)

Figure 5.10
Multidimensional adaptive filtering (180° MAF) permits a reduction of the noise level without significantly affecting the resolution. Excessive noise and streaks in the original reconstructions (upper row) are removed or reduced efficiently by preprocessing of the rawdata (lower row).

also serve to limit the dose: through z-filtering and the retrospective variation of the effective slice thickness, both images with high 3D spatial resolution and low-noise images for low-contrast evaluation can be provided without the need for additional exposure to radiation (see figure 4.16).

5.4.2 Technical Measures and New Approaches

Technical measures are known which improve the dose efficiency of CT systems and have been partly tested. However, their use often creates a conflict in relation to other goals and requirements. For example, increasing the filtration, which in fact does reduce the patient dose, requires higher mAs values and thus leads to greater loading of the x-ray tube. This in turn can lead to a limitation of the permissible scan duration for spiral CT (see figure 2.5). Multi-slice CT systems drastically reduce the scan duration, and the resulting reserves should also be utilized in connection with the use of additional filtration.

The definition and preparation of low-dose scanning protocols for pediatric CT and for special indications should be studied further and actively promoted by the manufacturers. The further development of noise-reducing reconstruction methods also appears to be promising, especially with regard to multidimensional adaptive filtering for multi-slice CT systems, which offer considerable potential [Kachelrieß, 1999]. The possibility shown in figure 5.10 for reducing noise without loss of spatial resolution can of course also be used for scanning at reduced dose while keeping the noise level unchanged.

A significant reduction of dose can also be achieved through an anatomy-adapted, that is an attenuation-dependent, tube current modulation [Gies, 1999; Kalender, 1999b,c]. The basic idea here is illustrated in figure 5.11a. The pixel noise in a CT image is largely attributable to the projections in which the greatest attenuation and therefore the greatest quantum noise occurs. This means that for cross-sections deviating significantly from a circular shape the intensity of the radiation can be reduced in the projections with less attenuation, without any significant effect on the noise pattern. This offers considerable potential for the reduction of dose without a deterioration of image quality, as can be seen clearly in figure 5.11b,c for an elliptical phantom. The dose reduction of about 50 % in this case has no visible effect on noise and image quality.

The human anatomy practically always shows cross-sections which deviate more or less significantly from a circular or cylindrical shape. Accordingly, the examinations with this technique (implemented as the work in progress CareDose package on Siemens SOMATOM PLUS 4 and Volume Zoom scanners) show that the mAs product can be reduced by typically between 10 % and 50 % without any loss of image quality. For scans with extreme differences in the attenuation characteristics between the a.p. and lateral directions, such as in the shoulder region, savings of even more than 50 % are possible [Greess, 1999; Kalender, 1999c]. With the use of tube current modulation, it is also possible to selectively influence image quality. Increasing the tube current in the lateral direction and reducing the current in the a.p. direction can improve the image quality and at the same time significantly reduce the dose; for the examination in figure 5.10d,e an mAs reduction of 32 % was achieved through increasing the current by 33 % in the lateral direction and reducing the current by 80 % in the a.p. direction. The actual patient dose is reduced even more strongly than the mAs product. In hip examinations, for example, we found typical values of mAs reduction around 40 %. As determined by phantom measurements [Kalender, 1999c] and by Monte Carlo calculations, these corresponded to a reduction in patient dose of 60 to 70 % (figure 5.12).

Spiral CT is predestined for this novel technique, since the required reference data for modifying the tube current are available in the shortest possible times and over the shortest possible distances. In our system, the currently used modulation parameters are determined in real-time from the immediately preceding values, taken from the oppositely located tube position, i.e. shifted by only 180° or half the table feed per rotation.

Alternative approaches, such as the "Smart Scan" procedure promoted by GE Medical Systems [Kopka, 1995a], make use of survey radiographs in the a.p. and lateral directions, but have so far been less successful. This is understandable, since the attenuation values are known for only two projec-

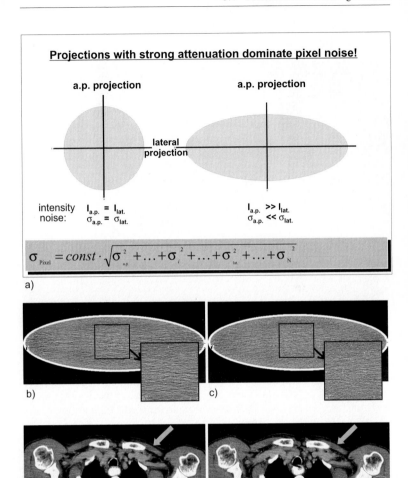

Figure 5.11
Anatomy-adapted tube current modulation.
Image noise is largely attributable to the projections in which the radiation is most
strongly attenuated **(a)**. By adapting the intensity to the attenuation, for the same dose
level the noise can be significantly reduced – **(b)** constant tube current, **(c)** modulated tube
current – or for the same noise level the dose can be reduced, for example by 32 % in **(d, e)**
[Kalender, 1999c].

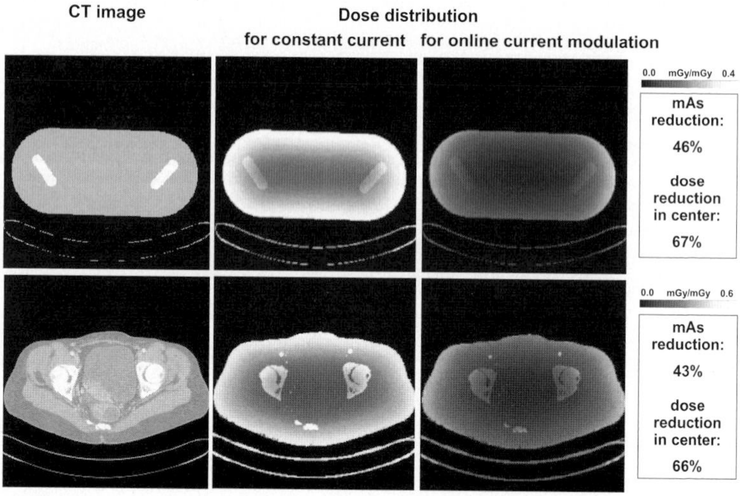

CT image   **Dose distribution**
        for constant current for online current modulation

Figure 5.12
Patient dose is reduced by tube current modulation. even more strongly than is indicated
by the mAs reduction (right column). This was confirmed both by measurements and
Monte Carlo calculations for phantoms and for patient studies.

tion directions and are approximated by a sinusoidal function. Furthermore,
operation is more difficult and requires a certain minimum of patient cooperation. Spiral CT offers substantially better and more practically oriented
prerequisites for anatomy-dependent tube current modulation.

5.5   Conclusions

The frequency of CT examinations has continued to increase in recent
years, in spite of the widespread availability of MR imaging. Thanks to the
newest technical developments, it is not expected that this trend will
reverse in the foreseeable future. On the contrary, the very possibilities
which multi-slice spiral CT offers will lead to a further increase in the
number of CT examinations performed. Consequently, it also appears to be
certain that the cumulative exposure of the population at large will remain
at the present level or increase. Since conventional radiography is used less
frequently, the relative contribution of CT to the yearly exposure of the
population at large to ionizing radiation for medical diagnoses will continue to increase. This represents a rational assessment of the ongoing
trend, without any intent to judge this situation.

A meaningful assessment can take place only if, along with the discussion
of possible risks, the clinical benefits, that is diagnostic reliability, patient
comfort, costs, etc. are also taken into consideration. Such a discussion

would go beyond the framework of the present book. In general, the benefits of CT examinations are not open to question. With regard to risks, on the other hand, there are widely different views held. It is of particular interest to me personally to enrich this discussion through the presentation of factual information and to contribute specific recommendations towards a possible consensus.

Here it is necessary to recognize two problems:

- The public is generally insecure concerning the question of the risks entailed in the use of ionizing radiation. The level of any particular exposure dose is usually not known.

- The public perceives that the cumulative dose per person within the population due to medically indicated exposures is increasing and that CT contributes a large part of this. Furthermore, it is known that the dose for a given examination can vary strongly from unit to unit and from user to user.

As a result, patients, but also the medical staff in many cases, are insecure and feel overburdened. An approach to a solution should follow two strategic directions:

- Optimization of CT systems and quality control. It must be assured that a definite level of image quality is obtained with a minimum dose.

- Information about CT dose values, but also information about benefits and risks. This information must be addressed equally to the staff, the patient and the broad public.

Approaches are already available and will be discussed at greater length below. Nevertheless, the commitment to their implementation requires further work, as well as achieving a consensus and formulations in standards and regulatory texts. The regulations for dose which have been required by the European lawmakers can contribute to this if they are implemented suitably.

5.5.1 Optimization of CT Systems and Quality Control

The optimization of CT systems with respect to image quality and dose efficiency has already been discussed. The support and guidance of the operating staff, for example through predefined scanning protocols, is no new demand and as such represents no new challenge. The already known measures must be supplemented by two further steps, which require the close cooperation of manufacturers and users:

- development of an automatic exposure control for CT and

- objectively defined requirements for image quality.

The combination of these two measures seeks to achieve and secure as its goal a definite level of image quality, attainable with minimum dose for the particular examination type. This would also define standards and reference dose values.

5.5.1.1 Automatic exposure control for CT

The developments in the direction of an anatomy-dependent, attenuation-based x-ray tube current modulation have shown a high potential for dose reduction [Greess, 1999; Kalender, 1999b; Kalender, 1999c]. These methods should be used on a broad basis, since they do not entail any disadvantages in terms of image quality. Their introduction on a general basis, however, should only represent a first step, because they are so far limited to the optimum distribution of a predefined mAs product per 360° revolution. A further necessary step must be the development of an automatic exposure control (AEC) for CT. Automatic exposure controls have long since become established in conventional x-ray diagnostics, although less for the purpose of dose reduction than for the prevention of faulty exposures. In CT the idea of an automatic dose control has not yet been followed up because, as a result of the prevailing high dynamic range of the receptor system, faulty exposures in the classical sense can be ruled out and because certain technical questions remained to be clarified.

These technical possibilities, such as the example of an anatomy-dependent tube current modulation, are in the meantime available. The remaining technical problem for the implementation of an AEC lies in the fact that, along with the regulation of the tube current during a 360° revolution, the tube current-time product – that is, the mAs value per revolution – has to be adapted continuously during a spiral CT examination to the changing body cross-section and the particular attenuation. This is technically feasible, provided that certain boundary conditions are considered, such as limitation of the maximum tube current. The essential problem is to arrive at an objective prescription of the image quality, for example in terms of image noise and image sharpness, required for a specific examination type. The problem which then results, to calculate the necessary tube current values from the measured CT data in real time, can be solved. The requirements for image quality must, however, first be defined from the radiological side.

5.5.1.2 Objectively defined requirements for image quality

Objective measures of image quality were defined and discussed in chapter 4. Nevertheless, experience shows that this cannot lay claim to a complete description of images. The subjective interpretation of images by the radiologist can very easily differ from an objectively determined order of ranking. This refers, for example, to noise patterns, which can be influenced by both the dose and the choice of convolution kernel. In spite of this, it should be possible to arrive at a consensus with respect to the decisive parameters, above all for image sharpness and noise.

This image quality, which is to be seen as the "minimum necessary" or, in the sense of radiation protection, as the "optimum" image quality for a particular application, must be ensured for all patients and without exception for all sections of the volume to be examined, with minimum dose. The dose would then automatically be reduced for the examination of a slender patient. This of course applies in special measure to pediatric CT, where minimum dose with the assurance of acceptable image quality is a matter of greatest importance. The dose would likewise be automatically reduced when, in the course of an examination, thinner cross-sections are reached, which is almost never realized under the conditions prevailing today.

A consensus concerning the required image quality parameters for commonly performed CT examinations would also improve the frequently criticized situation that different institutions work with substantially different parameters and consequently with radically different dose values. Differences of more than a factor of four have frequently been reported. This would also simplify the comparison of different CT scanners with regard to their dose requirements and enable the definition of acceptance criteria for general use.

Arriving at a consensus within a short time is desirable, but not necessarily to be expected. The concrete stipulations required for the operation of an automatic dose control can in principle be defined by and for any single particular user and be taken into consideration in an automatic exposure control. This alone would already represent a major step forward in the sense of a dose reduction.

5.5.2 Information about Dose, Benefits and Risks

Justified questions about dose values and also about the risks of an x-ray examination are often answered with great uncertainty, imprecision or not at all, and this can by itself contribute further to insecurity and suspicion. This is not at all necessary, and it is a simple matter to introduce improvements here. The program introduced for the calculation of patient dose in CT (see section 5.3.2), for example, is intended precisely to improve this situation. The specification of the patient dose for every CT examination, as mentioned at the beginning, will be required from CT manufacturers within the scope of implementing the EU patient directive. This is entirely meaningful, because information and transparency can also foster trust.

Peak dose values lie typically in the range of 5 to 50 mSv, and the effective dose in the range of 1 to 10 mSv. A positive aspect of estimating dose values when selecting the scan parameters or performing the examination is that behavior possibly specific to particular scanning modes, such as detector-side collimation with very thin slices, inadequate focus-side collimation with MSCT or the use of high-resolution combs, as well as their influence on the dose, immediately become more transparent for the user.

Particular attention is required for multiple examinations, dynamic CT and interventional CT, which however make up only a small percentage of the total number of CT examinations and for which the examination volume is often relatively small. At present the dose quantity which lawmakers will define as binding remains an open question. Here, it is desirable that patient-oriented parameters, such as the organ dose or effective dose, always be given in addition to the technical parameters required, such as – most likely – the dose length product.

The increased dissemination of information is entirely necessary, because it is astounding and often thoroughly disillusioning to see which news and statements, which speculations and conjectures, concerning dose and its effects are widely circulated in the media: "each single ray can kill!" and "thirty thousand cancer-related deaths per year from x-rays!" are typical reports finding echo in the German press; the fear of radiation, which arose during the time of the Cold War and with a view to the use of nuclear energy in its most destructive form has been transferred to the medical field.

Is it really true that each single ray may be lethal? All too often, reports and facts not likely to arouse sensationalism, but which would instead enable the patient and all concerned to assess the situation somewhat more neutrally and rationally, are given no consideration. Many facts and examples can be cited here:

- The average person carries more than 9,000 Becquerel of naturally occurring isotopes within the body. This translates to more than 9,000 radiogenic decay processes per second, more than 30 million per hour, and nearly a billion per day: suffice it to say, radiation is a part of our natural surroundings!

- All epidemiological studies which set out to prove that increased levels of natural radiation must inevitably lead to a higher incidence of cancer arrived at negative results. In most cases, just the opposite result was found. In the seven states of the USA, for example, which were shown to have double the normal level of natural radiation found in the rest of the USA, the incidence of cancer-related deaths was actually 15 % lower.

- The reports concerning the survivors of the atomic bombs dropped on Hiroshima and Nagasaki constitute the most important data for estimating the risk due to exposure to ionizing radiation [UNSCEAR, 1994]. While there can be no doubt that high dose values in fact led to an increased incidence of cancer-related deaths, it remains largely unnoticed that for dose values below 200 mSv this was not the case. With regard to the number of cases of leukemia, for example, the evaluation of which can be viewed as completed, since no further cases are to be expected here, in the range of 200 mSv there was in fact a significant reduction in the number of deaths among those exposed.

- A study of dockyard workers in the USA showed that for the 29,000 workers in the nuclear field, with the highest cumulative dose values, there was a lower incidence of cancer than for the non-nuclear control group comprising 33,000 of the same age and undergoing identical medical supervision. The difference was found to be 24%, in favor of the exposed workers, with a standard deviation of 16% [Matanoski, 1991].

The interesting and, at the same time disheartening, aspect of this is that results of this type remain largely ignored, while pure speculation is widely circulated. It is hardly necessary to think what would have appeared in the press if the death rate among the exposed workers had been 24% higher than for the control group. The fact that slightly increased radiation levels do not lead to any measurable negative effects is simply not sufficiently newsworthy.

We are certain that, with a high level of exposure, damage is probable and, with a very high dose, occurs beyond any doubt. In the low dose region, on the other hand, the corresponding data are lacking. All available sources indicate that extrapolation from the high dose region is not justified. The officially recognized assumption [ICRP, 1990] that the dose-effect relationship is strictly linear and that no threshold exists – the "linear, no threshold" (LNT) hypothesis – was formulated largely in the interest of safety consciousness, since no relevant data were available. In view of what is known today, however, this hypothesis must be seriously questioned [Jawarowski, 1999; Simmons, 1999; Mossman, 1998]

Already in the 1980s, results of studies in radiation biology were reported which reproducibly demonstrated that in the low dose region there are positive effects to be expected from exposure to radiation. A comprehensive review of such observations was published by Luckey [Luckey, 1982]. In the meantime, the results of a number of additional basic investigations have become available, which classify the basic effects observed. It can be assumed that in the region of low dose, up to about 500 mSv, several effects synergistically influence cell survival in a positive way and thus, up to 200 mSv, more than compensate for the harmful effects which occur at the same time (figure 5.13). Biopositive effects shown to take place for low-dose radiation were the detoxification of radicals from the cells, the removal and lessening of DNA damage and the activation of genes; a current summary, listing the numerous original studies, was recently given in [Feinendegen, 1999]. The negative effects, inducing cell damage, are not questioned in this model; at the same time, the positive effects are also considered. This also enables us to explain the numerous and apparently contradictory observations between low and high dose. These results and conclusions must be intensively discussed and evaluated at greater length, because they indicate that – for radiation also – the old principle might well apply: Solis dosis facet venenum – it is only the dose which makes the poison!

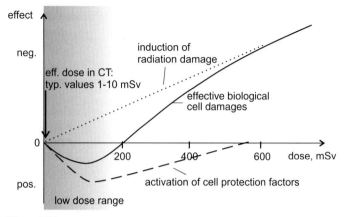

Figure 5.13
For the negative effects of ionizing radiation, a linear dose-effect relationship is generally assumed. Newer results indicate, however, that in the region up to about 200 mSv these effects are compensated for by biopositive effects [Feinendegen, 1999].

5.5.3   The Author's Summing up and Recommendations

The discussion concerning dose in CT will remain controversial. A consensus is certainly not in sight, which is why I would like to label the following summary as a personal statement. It is my intention to contribute factual information to the ongoing discussion. My motivation is the result of having frequently observed that patients are not only insecure, but react with fear.

It is entirely clear and proven beyond any doubt that a high dose of ionizing radiation can cause damage, which in extreme cases can result in death. It is just as certain, however, that there is little justification for the classification of CT as a "high dose examination procedure". The peak dose values lie as a rule in the range below 100 mSv, which is to say in the low dose range, for which it is not possible at present to make any definite statements.

As for the insecurity and the occasional panic which results from a purely irrational fear of radiation, a fear which is unfortunately widespread today, it is essential that accurate information be offered, precisely and above all for the benefit of the patient, who in many cases is largely insecure. The reference to the natural human environment would appear to be the most suitable and easiest to communicate. For this reason, I support the suggestion of Cameron [Cameron, 1991] to express dose values as multiples of the natural background radiation, with reference to the BERT (background equivalent radiation time) unit. Such means of expressing the dose would go a long way toward offering the uninitiated a classification of a particular dose value according to order of magnitude. This classification has already been implemented in the program WinDose [Kalender, 1999a], using the value of 2.4 mSv per year which applies for Germany. For the USA, the corresponding value is 3.0 mSv per year. Also, it is in fact correct and should be pointed out that the body is capable of sustaining repair mechanisms against damage caused by ionizing radiation.

The specification of the effective dose in BERT should offer an objectively understandable comparison. It conveys the fact that, in most cases, the dose in CT is of the order of magnitude of the yearly exposure arising due to natural background radiation. The individual organ dose values should also be specified in the same way. By definition, for partial body exposures these lie higher than the values for the effective dose.

Along with the yearly exposure due to natural background radiation of 2.4 mSv for Germany or 3.0 mSv for the USA, which is the most important reference value for the patient, the value 200 mSv may also be mentioned here, since this is very likely the value below which the natural resistance and repair mechanisms of the human body are able to reduce the probability of damage (figure 5.13). With modern CT technology, it appears to be possible to ensure that – with the exception of interventional procedures and dynamc CT – this value is never reached at any point in the body. The precautionary measures outlined above should in fact ensure that the dose values remain well below this value. The urgently recommended calculation of the values for the organ dose and effective dose would not only sharpen the awareness of dose, but can also serve to rule out the possibility of exceeding this value. If this value is exceeded, as might be necessary in special cases, this should at least be signaled. For the examination of infants and children, this concept should be implemented with particular thoroughness, with still further reduced upper limits. Such efforts and investigations are already in progress at the IMP in Erlangen.

It is therefore not my intention to in any way question radiation protection in general or in particular as this applies to CT. On the contrary, my efforts have been directed towards reducing the dose level for CT – see for example figures 5.10 to 5.12.

My intention is, in fact, to strengthen such efforts further and to make dose-related information available. This information can be used as a control and to support efforts to limit the dose level. This information should make clear that, for the realistic dose values discussed, the risk to the patient can be seen as negligibly small. The immense benefits of CT diagnosis to the patient, on the other hand, are certainly sufficiently known.

6 Processing and Visualization of Images

CT images, in most cases a complete batch of images, are available in digital form and – contrary to classical analog radiographs – can be processed directly by computer algorithms. The determination of density values, histograms and other tissue parameters, as well as geometric values, is possible at any time. Based on the original images, images can be generated in arbitrary orientation in two or three dimensional displays to provide appropriate views. Such evaluation and visualization approaches will be described in this chapter. As a supplement and for illustration purposes, the CD-ROM provides image examples, video clips and a software package for image display and evaluation. For CT novices, but also for all those who have so far viewed CT images mostly on film, interactive manipulation of image volumes may offer a better feeling for the possibilities given by modern CT imaging. Chapter 7 will allude to advanced image processing approaches, such as the automatic determination of lung or bone tissue compartments in special applications.

6.1 Simple Image Processing and Evaluation Procedures

Simple evaluation steps and possibilities for image manipulation are routine in CT. Among these are:

- determination of CT values of arbitrary pixels in the image
- determination of CT value profiles along arbitrary lines in the image
- choice of ROIs (circular, elliptical, rectangular, polygonal, ...)
- measurement of mean values and standard deviations for ROIs
- determination of CT value histograms for ROIs
- measurement of areas and volumes
- measurement of distances and angles
- magnification of image parts and panning
- filtering of images and
- addition, subtraction or other combinations of images.

Measurements with respect to geometry and density are required routinely. Distances, areas, volumes and angles are the geometric parameters most often asked for; in principle, this is simply an extension of measurements which are also carried out on conventional radiographs. The accuracy is much higher in CT, however, since no superposition problems exist and since CT offers the advantage of a distortion-free display, independently of the variable magnification factors given in radiography. For the assessment of tissue density, it is necessary to determine the mean value of a defined region of interest; in most cases the standard deviation, as a measure of homogeneity, is also determined. It can be supplemented by a display of the histogram of all CT values and respective parameters.

Most of the evaluation steps listed above are routinely available on CT consoles or independent evaluation stations; however, they are mostly still limited to single images. An extension and an improvement of evaluation has to include the third dimension in order to take account of volume scanning. It is obvious that distances and angles should be determined by using anatomical reference points in the 3D scan volume. Single images offer representative values of limited value. Only 3D evaluations can provide the correct geometrical result, since reference points are hardly ever in one single slice. Just the same, density measurements should be carried out for the complete lesion or organ of interest, i.e. for the complete 3D volume ('volume of interest' – VOI) instead of a 2D region. An evaluation of this type is usually carried out slice by slice by manual insertion or adaptation of ROIs. Methods of image processing for automated determination of such volumes of interest will bring about significant improvements in the future, since they relieve the user of a tedious job and they provide increased objectivity and reproducibility of the evaluation process (see also section 7.2).

6.2 Two-dimensional Displays

A CT image offers a two-dimensional display of the attenuation values in the imaged slice. In principle, each image shown in this chapter – no matter what it displays – is two-dimensional. The attributes two-dimensional (2D) and three-dimensional (3D) refer to the content of the image; i.e. 2D refers to displays of 2D distributions or slices and 3D to displays of complete 3D distributions or volumes.

Contrary to magnetic resonance tomography, CT scanning is primarily limited to the transverse plane as the direct scan plane. Only for the head and the extremities can scans be obtained directly in sagittal or coronal orientation with special positioning techniques. In most cases, however, it is necessary to synthesize such views from the original images. This is by no means problematic, since a cube of image data is always available, for spiral CT often in nearly isotropic resolution. In the simplest case, an image in sagittal or coronal orientation is built up by stringing together the same image row or line from a series of successive transverse images (figure 6.1). Images can be selected in arbitrary orientation; arbitrarily formed surfaces, oriented along anatomical structures, can also be generated. In general, these are called multiplanar reformations (MPR).

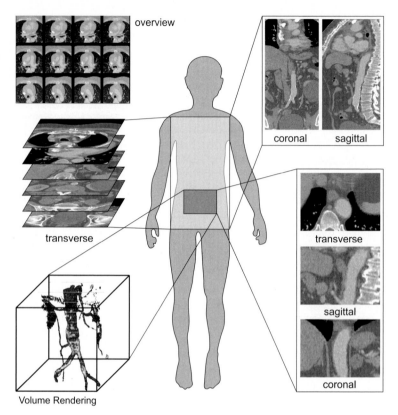

Figure 6.1
Various 2D display forms
A CT examination always provides an image data cube. In addition to single or multiple images (upper left), arbitrary reformations (right) can be generated. Contrary to 3D displays (lower left) 2D displays always represent the original CT values.

Interactive monitor viewing and evaluation of image volumes, here labeled iMPR in order to emphasize their interactive character, are controlled by moving a mouse or another input device. The operator may – similar to moving the transducer in ultrasound – approach anatomical structures or pathological details and, by moving back and forth slowly, select the slice or MPR where the detail of interest is displayed best, e.g. with highest contrast or largest diameter. This diagnostic approach is in the meantime generally available; especially four-quadrant displays with axial, sagittal, coronal and oblique slices offer a particularly good overview. The CD-ROM includes examples of these as exercises.

An extension of MPR techniques consists of generating arbitrarily thick slices ('slabs') from thin slices, reducing the noise level and possibly also improving the visualization of structures, for example vessels present in several slices. Preferably, this evaluation is carried out interactively also: using the mouse the thickness and the position of slabs can be defined and modified. The term 'sliding thin slab' (STS) is known for this technique, with iSTS-MPR or iSTS-MIP [Napel, 1993], respectively, indicating the interactive forms.

All the 2D displays mentioned have the particular advantage that CT values are presented directly and are not manipulated. Effects due to possible interpolations or calculation of mean values over several slices for STS approaches are negligible here. A simple orientation within the volume and an unambiguous interpretation of the pixel values is always given. Interactive evaluation at the monitor is the approach which allows viewing and diagnosing the large image data volumes accumulating today in a convenient and efficient manner. Documenting images on film first and then reading the films does not constitute an alternative anymore in view of the cost of film and the handling problem (see section 6.4). An interactive selection of subvolumes of interest (figure 6.1) and the use of 3D display methods are further steps which follow directly in monitor viewing.

6.3   Three-dimensional Displays

Three-dimensional displays serve to represent the scan volume in only one image with a high degree of faithfulness and accentuate the diagnostically relevant details. This can be done successfully to a high degree when only one structure, for example the skeleton or contrast medium-filled vessels have to be displayed, i.e. whenever structures with high contrast in relation to their surroundings are concerned. The original CT value information is lost, however. The different procedures display, for example, only surfaces (shaded surface displays – SSD) or maximum CT values (maximum intensity projections – MIP). So-called volume rendering (VR) techniques, including near-realistic endoscopy-like displays of internal body structures, known as perspective volume renderings (pVR), allow more flexible forms of volume displays. These approaches will be explained in detail in the following sections.

All forms of 3D displays require the user to select an observer position for which the computer will render the given 3D data volume. A two-dimensional image oriented normal to the viewing direction is calculated point by point. To build up such a display, all CT values along each ray from the observer through the 3D data volume to each image point have to be taken into account and entered with appropriate weighting factors. The CT value profile of the central search ray through the subvolume selected in figure 6.1 lower left is therefore shown schematically in each of the following figures and is used for illustration purposes. All 3D displays can be built up as a central projection or as a parallel projection. Central projections are preferred for SSD, VR and pVR and parallel projections for MIP.

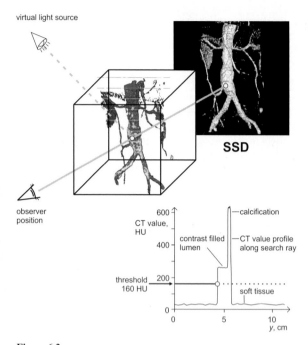

Figure 6.2
Threshold-based surface display
The voxel along a search ray from an assumed observer position through the 3D data volume is determined for which a predefined CT value is reached or exceeded for the first time. A surface is computed taking all determined points into account and is illuminated to generate shading effects.

6.3.1   Surface Displays

In most forms of surface renderings, the user has to select a threshold CT value. For each search ray from the observer position through the given 3D data volume to the image plane, the particular voxel is determined for which the given threshold value is reached or exceeded for the first time. In figure 6.2 this is the case when the search ray reaches the contrast medium-filled vessel lumen, i.e. when the threshold value of 160 HU chosen here is exceeded for the first time along the CT value profile. In the simplest case, the distance of this point to the observer position can be displayed coded as a gray value. For surface shaded displays, a surface is reconstructed using all the available points and a computation is carried out to determine how much light emitted by a fictitious light source is reflected by each surface point, depending on the surface orientation (figure 6.2). Displays of this type generate a largely realistic three-dimensional impression. The shading effects created gave rise to the term 'shaded surface displays' which is commonly used.

Several limitations and pitfalls may result for SSDs. When several structures which exceed the given threshold values are superimposed in the viewing direction, only the structure closest to the observer will be visible; all structures behind it, although possibly exhibiting much higher CT values, will remain hidden. To display such structures either a different viewing direction has to be chosen or the structure responsible for the hiding has to be removed from the data volume by editing. The biggest problem with SSDs, however, is given by the dependence of the generated display on the predefined threshold value. The wall thickness of bony structures or vascular stenoses, for example, can be manipulated arbitrarily by lowering and raising the threshold value. Raising the threshold will result in bone defects ('fenestration') and higher degrees of stenosis; lowering the threshold can cause the display of pixels with CT values increased due to noise fluctuations ('flying pixels') and stenoses can be hidden. This implies that surface shaded displays are not suitable for diagnostic purposes. SSDs are utilized most often to document the diagnostic finding; displays of bony structures are the most important field of this application.

6.3.2 Projection Displays

For maximum intensity projections (MIP) the point, i.e. the voxel, with the highest CT value along the search ray from the observer to the image plane is determined. This value is displayed directly in the image (figure 6.3); a minimum of CT value information is thereby preserved. This implies that a given MIP image is simply a 2D projection image. A 3D impression, which is not generated intentionally in the MIP procedure, can be deceptive. To accentuate the spatial relationships a series of MIP images can be generated by incrementing the viewing direction in small steps and viewing these images in a cine loop.

As an alternative to the pixels with highest intensity, projection images can be generated which display the lowest intensities; such images, often called MinIP, can be useful, for example, to display the bronchial tree. The summation of all voxel values along the search ray and appropriate scaling produces images similar to classical radiographs. Contrary to radiographs, however, such CT-based projection displays can be limited to an organ or partial subvolume of interest which can be selected arbitrarily (figure 6.1).

6.3.3 Volume Rendering Displays

Volume visualization and volume rendering can be considered synonyms; rendering is a term taken from computer graphics and represents the process of generating a 2D image from a 3D model. VR approaches are superior to the previously discussed SSD and MIP procedures both in the fundamental approach and with respect to performance. For each search ray from the eye of the observer to the resulting image pixels all voxels may contribute to the resulting image by using adequate weighting, instead of

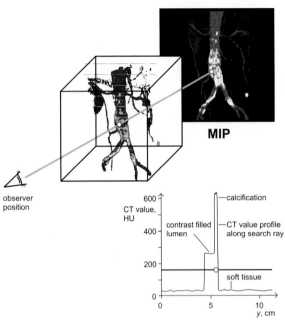

Figure 6.3
Maximum intensity projections
The maximum CT value found along each search ray from the observer through the 3D
data volume to the fictitious image plane is used directly for display.

only a single voxel. Selectable and interactively modifiable transfer functions allow the assignment of opacity and color to each CT value (figure 6.4). For example, normal soft tissue can be assigned high transparency, contrasted vessels slight opaqueness and bone strong opaqueness. Color is additionally used in most cases, with the color intensity decreasing with increasing distance to the observer in order to generate depth information and a 3D impression.

Transfer functions can be generated or selected in such a way that the resulting image resembles a shaded surface display. However, it is much more interesting and desirable in most cases to present 3D anatomy, for example the vascular tree, in a clear manner without removing the surrounding anatomy completely.

Volume rendering is considered the method of choice among the 3D rendering approaches, due to its great variability of display possibilities and to the attractive images which it generates. It should be mentioned, however, that training and experience are required in order to obtain successful results and that higher demands are imposed on hardware and software. Volume rendering for large data sets, e.g. more than 500 images in a 512

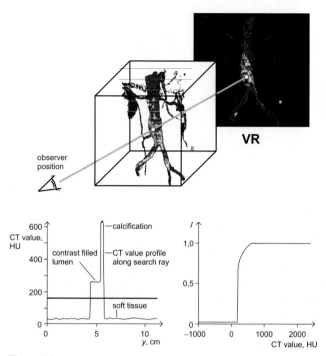

Figure 6.4
Volume rendering
Opacity and color are assigned to each CT value interval via so-called transfer functions. The sum of all CT values along each search ray from the observer through the 3D data volume, weighted by the transfer functions, is displayed. Color intensities are used to enhance the 3D impression.

× 512 matrix, is not yet available in real time. However, it is only a question of time until we will have this at our disposal.

6.3.4   Virtual Endoscopy

Perspective volume rendering represents a dedicated form of the volume rendering technique described above, which aims at providing virtual endoscopic views. The predominant field of application for this technique, the so-called virtual endoscopy (VE), is the diagnostic evaluation of anatomical structures which are also amenable to endoscopes; these are, for example, the bronchial tree, the larger vessels, the colon and the paranasal sinus system. In addition to these common applications virtual endoscopy can be used in areas such as the brain cisterns and in the gastrointestinal region, which are not directly accessible for endoscopes.

In general, a perspective view of the near environment of the endoscope's tip is required. The opacity and color functions are mostly selected in such

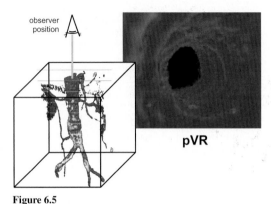

Figure 6.5
Perspective volume rendering
The display is generated similarly to volume rendering. However, a perspective view as seen by a camera placed close-by is generated using specially adapted opacity functions.

a way as to present the transition from intestinal, bronchial or vessel lumen etc. to the surrounding tissues, i.e. the intestinal wall, the bronchial wall or the vessel wall, respectively, with a high degree of opaqueness (figure 6.5). Often it is informative or diagnostically important to view the structures under motion and from different directions, similar to the way an endoscope or a surgical microscope is utilized. So-called 'fly throughs' through the volume can be generated, which provide the impression of a virtual flight through the selected body region. This is not only instructive and aesthetically appealing, but in many cases also diagnostically valuable. This has been shown in particular for virtual coloscopy [McFarland, 1997], bronchoscopy [Vining, 1996], and virtual cisternoscopy [Fellner, 1998]. An interesting aspect is often made possible as a result of a feature immanent to pVR, namely the possibility of viewing details from different directions, whereas real endoscopes can only produce images in the direction of their forward motion.

6.3.5   Recommendations on the Choice of 3D Display Methods

For the utilization of the various display forms there is a puzzling number of options and variations available. Table 6.1 gives an overview of the characteristics and parameters which are frequently used.

The literature includes a large number of publications on the different display approaches and their use for various diagnostic tasks, for example [Rubin, 1996; Blank, 2000]; some typical examples for applications are given in figure 6.6. The CD-ROM offers additional examples, in color and with animation.

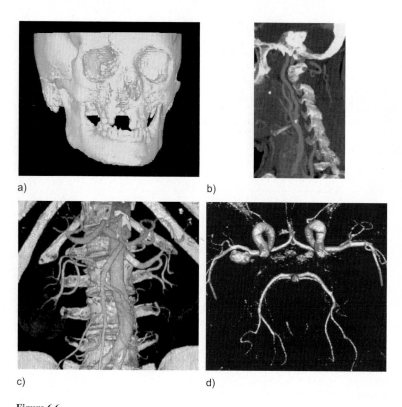

Figure 6.6
Examples for typical uses of the different 3D display methods
a) SSD for displaying skeletal structures.
b) MIP for CT angiography.
c) VR for viewing abdominal structures.
d) pVR for performing virtual cisternoscopy for preoperative planning.

All attempts to define the role and the performance of the various display forms suffer from the fact that the results and conclusions have to be reviewed continuously due to the steady technical progress and improved applicability. Volume rendering approaches, in particular, have not been widely available and are not easily practicable in all cases. We can safely assume that technical developments will provide enhanced performance, but also that various personal preferences will remain. My own expectation is that volume rendering with user-friendly, preset evaluation protocols will prevail as the method of choice in 3D display forms. However, they will only supplant and augment, but not replace 2D displays.

With respect to the choice between 2D and 3D displays, a simple tip may suffice in most cases: diagnosis has to be performed in the majority of cases by reviewing original images or multiplanar displays, i.e. using 2D

Table 6.1   Use of various parameters for 2D and 3D displays

	Color	Illumination	Perspective	Interaction, motion
MPR	no	no	no	yes
MIP	no	no	no	yes
SSD	no	yes	yes	yes
VR	yes	yes	no	yes
pVR	yes	yes	yes	yes

representations and the actual CT value information. The documentation of the findings, however, will be supported or solely provided by 3D displays, in particular when directed to the referring physician or surgeon. The reason for this distinction is that the original and MPR images represent the full and unperturbed CT value information, whereas 3D images allow an easy and clear overview. But many details in these views may be generated artificially or omitted arbitrarily due to the selected thresholds, transfer functions etc. or due to other effects.

6.4   How to Handle all the Images

High resolution in the third dimension is a specific advantage deriving from spiral CT and, even more so, from multi-slice spiral CT. This necessarily implies the scanning of large volumes with thin slice collimation and overlapping image reconstruction, i.e. it implies a large number of images. In the meantime, three digit numbers are the rule. The peripheral angiography shown on the book cover, for example, represents 570 images, and the aortography (figure 6.1 ff.) shown in this chapter represents 522 images. There is no upper limit. Not surprisingly, then, in many cases the first reaction to the use of MSCT in routine frequently is: How will we handle all the images?

Documentation on film or other hardcopy media and the subsequent reading of these media is hardly practical and certainly not up to date. The related costs also speak against this approach; a single sheet of film, for example, costs more than a CD-ROM. For the documentation of one of the cases mentioned above approximately 50 films would be required, while a single CD-ROM can hold this data volume without any problem. Thus, storage and archival should be performed in digital form for cost reasons alone. An additional and important advantage results from the fact that the complete information remains available and not only the gray values within the window chosen for the hardcopy.

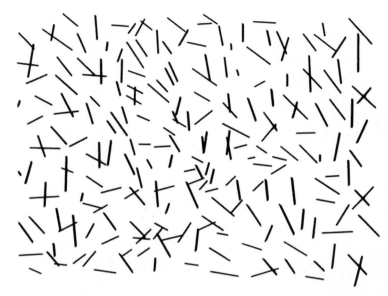

Figure 6.7
What kind of animal is hidden in this drawing? It can be easily recognized in the video clip 'motion.avi' on the CD-ROM when motion is activated. This phenomenon, improved recognition of moving objects, can be utilized in interactive viewing.

Reading of cases should be done interactively at the monitor of the CT unit or at a work station. In principle, then, the huge data volumes do not represent a problem, assuming that appropriate hardware and software are at hand. Technically, this no longer constitutes a problem today. More often the problem is linked to the organization and the management of processes. Having to part with film appears to be difficult for many radiologists.

For a simple demonstration that even large data volumes can be easily handled with today's technology, the enclosed CD-ROM offers an evaluation software package (ImpactView) which can run on arbitrary PCs or laptops under Windows 98 and Windows NT. If an appropriate memory size is available, the cases provided can be viewed interactively and, for example, be demonstrated via video beamer. In addition to the possibility of efficient presentation in clinical routine, such a software lends itself to other use, as for example in teaching or for presentations. The intention in connection with this textbook is to offer to the CT novices among the readers the possibility of familiarizing themselves with CT images and techniques and exploring the human anatomy interactively by browsing through some image sets. Teachers can use it in a similar way for demonstrations, independently of a CT console or an evaluation station. The use of iMPR, interactive four-quadrant MPR displays, is my specific recommendation for this.

A specific advantage of interactive viewing can be observed. The human visual system has specialized during the course of evolution in the recognition of moving objects or structures particularly well, for example the enemy or the predator suddenly appearing on the scene. In figure 6.7 an animal is hidden which, although not dangerous, nevertheless is not easily detected. Only when it moves is it recognized immediately. This can be understood by viewing the short video clip 'motion.avi' on the CD-ROM as soon as motion is initiated. The phenomenon that moving details are more easily recognized can be utilized for example when browsing through a lung volume. A solitary lung nodule appearing suddenly on the scene can be easily differentiated from the surrounding vascular and bronchial structures which remain quasi-static.

The question of whether a definite advantage for interactive case readings results remains to be investigated. Nevertheless, the practical advantages of monitor reading appear obvious. Contrary to the use of a film alternator, the complete volume can be easily accessed. Windowing, magnification and all evaluation and display functions discussed in this chapter are available without any limitations.

7 Special Applications

7.1 General Considerations

In the competition of modern imaging modalities – predominantly waged between CT, MR, PET and ultrasound – refinements of techniques and thereby also special applications have become more and more important. Often they may be taken as a measure for the degree of maturity and reliability of the method applied, and they may lead to broad clinical applications. Fast volume scanning by spiral CT, which initially constituted an exotic special application, is one example for such a development. CT angiography is another.

CT is used routinely from the head to the body trunk and the extremities for all body organs and anatomical regions, for patients of all sizes and age groups, covering pediatric to geriatric problems. There is no exact definition of what is a special application. They arise whenever additional technical equipment of the scanner, special scanning protocols or the availability of dedicated image processing or evaluation software is required, i.e. requirements beyond routine applications. Accordingly, the requirements with respect to the training of personnel are greater, and sometimes special applications are not compatible with routine operation.

The list of typical examples given below is intended to indicate the broad spectrum of special applications in CT, but by no means claims to be complete, since such a list may vary from institution to institution and is in any case subject to continuous change. Among the special applications are:

- CT angiography,

- Dynamic CT:
  assessment of contrast medium kinetics in different tissues
  measurement of brain perfusion
  measurement of myocardial perfusion

- Interventional CT

- Quantitative CT:
  bone density measurement
  lung density measurement
  coronary calcium measurement

- Phase-selective (4D) imaging of the heart.

CT angiography (CTA) is now widely used and therefore might also be considered a routine application. After intravenous injection of a contrast medium bolus, which provides the best possible vascular contrast for typically 30 to 40 seconds, the anatomic range of interest has to be scanned by spiral CT during exactly this period of time. The difficulty lies in the task of exactly matching the time windows for contrast enhancement and scanning, since the bolus arrival time may vary strongly from individual to individual. To ensure good results a test bolus can be injected to determine its arrival time by repeated scans of a single slice. Alternatively, the arrival of the actual bolus can be determined by sequential scans of a single slice and by switching to the volume scan after detecting its arrival as fast as possible [Kopka, 1995b]. This approach is supported by the manufacturers with options such as CareBolus and SmartPrep. While the timing of bolus and scan requires effort and experience, the 3D display and evaluation – using the methods described in the previous chapter – are becoming increasingly accessible. Image examples have already been shown and are also included on the CD-ROM.

Dynamic CT was already discussed with respect to the technical prerequisites in section 2.3.4. It serves to assess changes in attenuation with time. These may be caused by physiological processes, such as the beating of the heart or pulmonary respiration. In clinical applications the assessment of contrast medium kinetics in different body sections is most frequently required. To obtain this a representative section (respectively M sections for multi-slice scanners) or a volume is selected, the contrast medium is administered and the selected slice(s) or the selected volume scanned repeatedly. The requirements for temporal sampling depend on the physiological process in question and on the type of contrast medium: to assess brain tissue perfusion by measuring the accumulation of xenon during continuous inhalation of a xenon-oxygen mixture, for example, scans are typically taken over five to ten minutes at one-minute intervals (figure 7.1a, b).

The Kety equation provides an accepted physiological model, and the xenon method provides absolute values with high accuracy [Kalender, 1991c]. Nevertheless, "Xenon CT" has not been successful in the sense of a broad application, since a high degree of patient cooperation is demanded which cannot be fulfilled in clinical routine. Any type of movement during the examination leads to errors in the assessment of tissue perfusion. An alternative is given by recording the transit of a short contrast medium bolus applied intravenously with high temporal resolution over a short time [Miles, 1997]. Instead of single scans at larger time intervals, continuous scanning is used in most cases. Examinations of this type are carried out for patients with an acute stroke, for example, to decide on the type of therapy indicated by the remaining tissue perfusion measured with this method (figure 7.1c, d) [König, 1998]. Dynamic CT can and will be extended to further fields of application, for example to measuring myocardial or tumor perfusion.

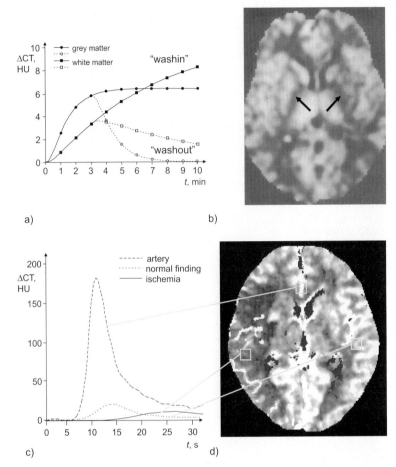

Figure 7.1
Dynamic CT can be performed with measurements in intervals of the order of magnitude of minutes (xenon inhalation (**a, b**) [Kalender, 1991c]) or seconds, respectively, (contrast medium bolus (**c, d**) [König, 1998]) to assess brain tissue perfusion.

Interventional CT comprises CT-guided or CT-controlled procedures such as punctures to obtain biopsies, drainages or numerous other therapeutical interventions. Mechanical means to position or to guide the instruments are often provided, supported by software to determine the target coordinates from CT images and to calculate the parameter sets for such devices. The specific demands on the CT scanner are dictated by the need to supervise the respective intervention in real time in many cases. Particularly in the body trunk, which may be subject to movements at any time, the intervention – for example the positioning of a puncture needle – has to be controlled continuously (figure 7.2). This serves to exclude the risk of damage

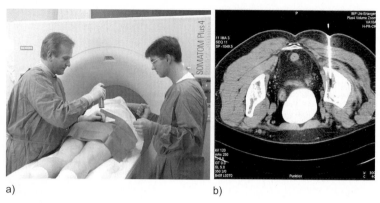

a)   b)

Figure 7.2
Interventional procedures, such as biopsies (**a**), can be performed safely under CT image
guidance and control (**b**).

to critical organs or structures, but also to control the success of a therapeutic intervention at any time and to permit adequate adjustments. For this reason the shortest possible scan times and reconstruction times are of utmost importance in interventional CT, as discussed in section 2.3.5. Whenever continuous imaging in near real-time is provided, one speaks of CT fluoroscopy. This is available today on most modern scanners with continuous scanning and capable of calculating several images per second.

The use of multi-slice scanning allows improved control of the target volume, since simultaneous scanning of several slices determines the position of the needle tip unambiguously and allows precise adjustment of the table position at any time. These technical capabilities are clearly welcome, since many minimally invasive interventions can then be carried out more easily and safely. However, the patient dose may increase significantly for longer interventions. Adequate software support for dose monitoring and measures to reduce dose, which are state of the art in conventional interventional fluoroscopy, are still in an early phase of development for CT at present.

7.2   Quantitative CT

The task of providing quantitative results, i.e. in our case quantitative CT (QCT), often makes the strictest demands on imaging modalities and provides a measure of the maturity and reliability of a particular modality or apparatus. Several QCT applications have already been mentioned. Quantitative results can be obtained by simple geometric measures, such as the size and volume of a tumor. But there are many more complex procedures, such as options to measure the bone mineral density, the calcium content

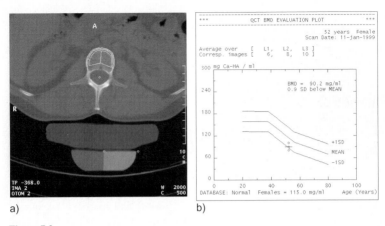

a)   b)

Figure 7.3
The determination of the density of spongious and cortical bone at the lumbar spine represents an established QCT procedure for which automated evaluation software (**a**), calibration phantoms and reference values (**b**) are available.

of the coronary arteries or the density and the structure of the lung. The
assessment of tissue perfusion by dynamic CT, which was discussed above,
is not necessarily a QCT application, since only perfusion patterns are
obtained as parameter images, but with no claim of absolutely quantitative
values. Accepted models and criteria to validate such values are still miss-
ing.

All statements of quantitative values require particular caution, since diagnostic or therapeutic decisions may potentially be based on a single determined number, and in any case they may be influenced by it. For example,
follow-up controls to assess tumor growth have to provide reliable measures of the volume to allow therapeutic decisions to be taken. Similarly,
the measurements of bone mineral density have to be precise whenever this
parameter is used for the follow-up of osteoporosis. There is no limit to the
number of examples which can be given to illustrate the potential importance of quantitative values and the requirements for particular care and for
quality assurance measures. The discussions following below will refer to
bone mineral density (figure 7.3) and to lung density measurements, both
of which have been introduced as QCT product options (OSTEO CT and
PULMO CT on the SOMATOM PLUS). Additionally, the QCT application
"coronary calcium scoring" will be discussed in the next section. Based on
these examples we will see that similar principles and considerations apply
to all QCT applications.

To judge the quality of a quantitative procedure in a technical and physical
sense the following criteria, which would hardly be questioned for standard
imaging, are of primary importance here:

- accuracy

- reproducibility or precision

- quality assurance and

- comparability with other scanners.

The accuracy of a measurement, i.e. the measure of how close the determined value comes to the true value, is often considered the most important criterion. For many medical applications, however, it is less relevant than the reproducibility. The assignment of "normal" or "diseased" based on a single quantitative value is often not possible, since nature has provided considerable variation in many parameters for human beings. For example, for the distribution of bone density in healthy individuals of the same age and sex a standard deviation of about 30% has to be considered typical (figure 7.2b). An accuracy of about 10% appears sufficient in this case; more stringent requirements, which would not be easy to fulfil, offer no significant advantage.

The reproducibility of the measurement is the parameter of greater importance in most cases, since it will determine if follow-up controls are meaningful. For example, the bone mineral density measurements mentioned above aim to distinguish with certainty between bone losses of 1 to 2% per year, which are still considered normal, and higher loss rates. To be able to reliably diagnose a loss of 5% requires a measurement reproducibility of better than 2%. Generally it must be said that a change in the patient's condition can only be assessed with statistical certainty if it exceeds 2.8 times the standard deviation ($2 \cdot \sqrt{2}$ or "3σ"rule). This implies that σ has to be one third or less of the minimum change to be measured. Such high precision can only be obtained with special effort.

For bone mineral measurements, taking the above into account, this means:

- An accuracy of 5 to 10% is considered sufficient and is possible using appropriate calibration procedures.

- A reproducibility of better than 2% is desirable. This requires establishing fixed scan protocols, automated evaluation procedures and calibration procedures.

- For quality assurance, a calibration standard has to be measured at least during monthly quality constancy testing, preferably along with each patient measurement.

- Comparability of results between different scanners is a prerequisite for establishing the general acceptance of an application. Again, an accepted calibration standard has to be defined and be used to achieve this goal.

The respective prerequisites, to give an example, are provided in the OSTEO CT option. Fixed scan protocols are preset, and automated objective evaluation procedures [Kalender, 1987c] and a calibration standard, referencing the European Spine Phantom [Kalender, 1995b], are included, together with age- and sex-matched reference data for a healthy population.

For quantitative CT of the lung, problems of measurement reproducibility are once again of primary concern, since considerable, mostly patient-related, variations can occur. Lung density varies greatly with the degree of inspiration; within the limits of vital capacity (VC) differences of more than a factor of 2 to 3 may result. A control of the depth of inspiration is therefore required to ensure adequate reproducibility and thus to allow for follow-up studies. Spirometric control appears to be the method of choice and offers the possibility to trigger the scan at a desired defined depth of inspiration [Kalender, 1990a]. For this purpose the patient has to breathe through a spirometer during the complete examination. Initially, a measurement of the vital capacity is carried out to determine a reference value. The CT scans can be taken at arbitrary values; 50% of VC is frequently selected, since this represents a comfortable level for the patient. In most cases only a few representative slices are measured with the carina, depicted in the a.p. survey radiograph used for orientation; however, volume scans by spiral CT can be obtained in the same way with this technique.

For QCT of the lung also, automated procedures should be used for the numerical evaluation of the images in order to improve reproducibility [Kalender, 1991a]. Similar to bony tissue, the lung also represents a very inhomogeneously structured organ. The placement of ROIs, in particular for regional evaluation, is therefore very critical. Automated algorithms not only allow for a reproducible evaluation using objectively defined criteria, but are also very fast and comfortable and they offer a great variety of evaluation parameters. Calibration and quality assurance in PULMO CT are based on an anthropomorphic phantom similar to the approach in bone mineral measurements.

The general conclusion, which is supported by many research and clinical groups, is that quantitative CT has to be supported by dedicated measures in any case. In the best case the appropriate measures are provided directly by the manufacturer, who is in a position to control all factors of influence. The respective demands also apply to the coronary calcium measurements discussed below if this application is to achieve a high quality standard and wide acceptance.

7.3   Cardiac Imaging and Coronary Calcium Measurements

It is generally expected that the heart can be imaged well if its structures do not move significantly during the time of the scan or, for retrospective approaches, during the effective scan time. For rotation times of 500 ms and for low heart frequencies this assumption is valid to a high degree for the diastolic phase, where phases of relatively little motion are given for 250 ms or more in many cases. For higher heart frequencies and for different motion phases of the heart, this assumption no longer holds true. Scan times of less than 50 ms would be required to image the heart in all phases of motion without any influence of motion [Ritchie, 1992].

The most straightforward approach is to image the complete heart consistently during the slow-motion diastolic phase, since the highest image quality can be expected in this case. This can be achieved with sequential CT, just as with electron beam CT, by scanning sequentially with prospective ECG triggering and partial scan acquisition. This approach is popular for coronary calcium measurements. In such single slice acquisitions, however, the total examination time frequently exceeds 30 s, leading to respiration-induced registration problems from slice to slice. Multi-slice acquisition and the spiral technique offer decisive advantages here. For this reason this complete section is focussed on retrospective ECG-correlated spiral CT reconstruction, which also allows phase-selective imaging in a simple manner. The required dedicated z-interpolation algorithms have already been introduced in section 3.4.3.

For cardiac CT application it is generally true that the table feed per heart beat should not exceed the total collimation width $M \cdot S$, where the time interval per heart beat follows directly from the heart frequency f_H. The maximum table speed is then

$$d' = \frac{M \cdot S}{1/f_H} \, , \tag{7.1}$$

the table feed per rotation

$$d \leq M \cdot S \cdot f_H \cdot t_{rot} \, . \tag{7.2}$$

and therefore the pitch is

$$p \leq \frac{d}{M \cdot S} = f_H \cdot t_{rot} \, . \tag{7.3}$$

This implies that for spiral CT of the heart the pitch is limited to relatively small values. For a rotation time of 0.5 s and a heart frequency $f_H = 60$ beats per minute (bpm) a maximum pitch of 0.5 results and for $f_H = 120$ bpm a maximum value of 1.0.

In addition to imaging of the heart in general and to CT coronary angiography, phase-selective displays of the heart and measurement of coronary calcium content are of particular interest and will be discussed below. None of the applications described is widely established at present. The very convincing image results which have been achieved up to now, strongly suggest that a complete new field of application for CT will develop. The high quality of results, as for example the display of a stenosis and of soft

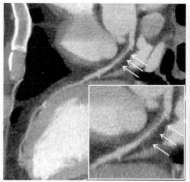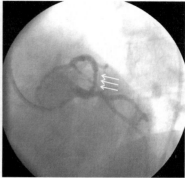

Figure 7.4
ECG-correlated image reconstruction with algorithm 180°MCI collects data from successive heart beats using a combined temporal filtering and z-filtering approach. The high
temporal resolution (down to less than 100 ms for a rotation time of 0.5 s) allows to accurately display the cardiac anatomy for all heart rates (up to 150 bpm and more). Here, the
display of a stenosis and of soft plaque (left) is demonstrated in direct comparison to conventional angiography (right).

plaque in figure 7.4, is also illustrated by examples on the CD-ROM, some
of these as animated video clips.

7.3.1   Phase-selective Imaging of the Heart with MSCT

Heart phase-selective imaging can in principle be realized by the repeated
prospective triggering of sequential scans or by ECG-correlated single-slice
spiral CT reconstructions. However, dose considerations and practical reasons speak against such solutions. Multi-slice spiral CT with subsecond
rotation times offers an astounding increase in potential here.

Partial scan reconstructions from MSCT scan data, which require an effective scan time of less than 300 ms for rotation times of 500 ms (see section
3.4.3), provide astonishingly good results (180°MCD). This is illustrated in
figure 7.5. in a direct comparison of the different approaches. While image
quality is generally limited for the standard 180°MLI reconstruction and
does not allow for phase selection, ECG-correlated reconstructions
obtained from the same data set with the 180°MCD and 180°MCI algorithms yield significant improvement. The first row for both cases in figure
7.5 shows a systolic image, the second row a diastolic image, and the third
row an MPR reconstruction for the diastolic phase again. For higher heart
frequencies, here by comparison of two cases with 51 bpm (top) and 95
bpm (bottom), limitations of 180°MCD become apparent, most clearly in
the multiplanar displays. These are only evident for higher heart frequencies, since here the diastolic phase is also shortened and falls below 250
ms. Such problems could be reduced or eliminated by a further reduction
of rotation times.

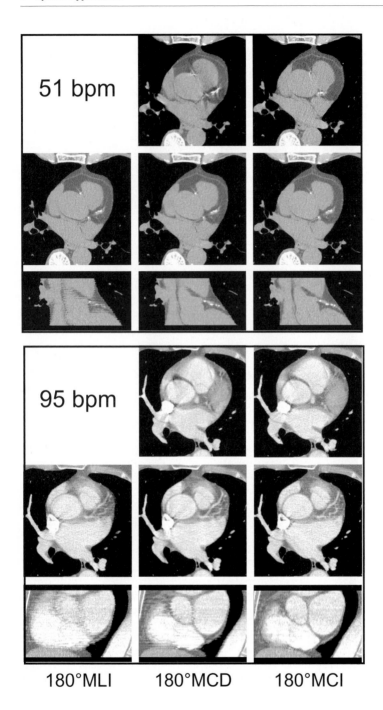

180°MLI   180°MCD   180°MCI

The special interpolation algorithm 180°MCI offers significant improvements with respect to temporal resolution, since only relatively short sections of the R-R interval are used. Depending on the relation of heart frequency and rotation frequency effective scan times of less than 100 ms can be reached [Kachelrieß, 2000b]. This allows for phase-selective displays of the heart even at higher pulse rates. As can be viewed in animation on the CD-ROM, these are quite impressive. It is difficult, however, to determine how sharp and how reliable such displays are for heart phases associated with fast motion. The clinical examples only allow a qualitative and subjective assessment. Simulation results and subjective impressions have been investigated and confirmed objectively by an experimental setup with a PC-controlled robot which simulates the three-dimensional motion of the heart during the scan; MSCT with a rotation time of 0.5 s using the 180°MCI algorithm can provide temporal resolution below 100 ms. The majority of manufacturers presently offer or prepare the 180°MCI approach in various implementations. Combinations of 180°MCD and 180°MCI, which adapt to the given heart frequency, represent an interesting hybrid approach currently being pursued by Siemens Medical Systems. The quality control tools discussed in the next section and shown in figure 7.6 will help to determine the optimal approach.

7.3.2   Coronary Calcium Measurements with CT

Coronary heart disease is the most frequent cause of death in our society. The search for non-invasive methods for an early and certain diagnosis and for reliable follow-up control continues. The detection of vascular stenosis is a method of choice; in addition to the established fluoroscopy-based coronary angiography, the development of a less invasive CT coronary angiography has become a highly relevant research topic. Calcifications of the coronary arteries, although not highly specific, are considered a further indicator for coronary heart disease. CT gives us the possibility to display calcifications and their three-dimensional distribution and to assess them quantitatively.

Coronary calcium measurements, which are often referred to as "coronary calcium scoring" in the literature, have been performed on EBCT scanners for many years (section 2.4.1). Nevertheless, the procedure cannot be considered mature or established. There are no statements on accuracy in clinical work; again, however, this parameter is less important, similar to bone density measurements. The reproducibility has been specified with approximately 30 % [Bielak, 1994]. Applying the "3σ" rule quoted above, this

◄ **Figure 7.5**
Comparison of results for standard reconstructions (180°MLI, left) and for ECG-correlated image reconstruction (180°MCD, center; 180°MCI, right)

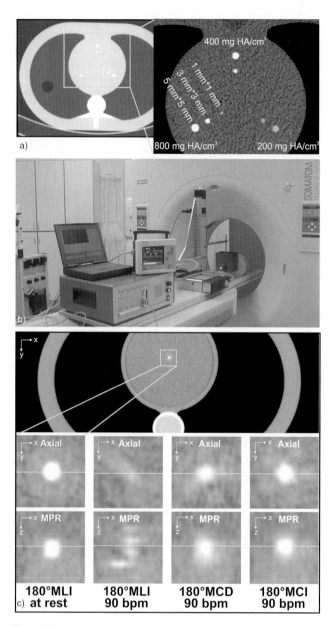

Figure 7.6
Quality control for coronary calcium measurements. An anthropomorphic thorax phantom with replaceable calibration inserts (**a.**) for static calibration and a motion phantom (**b.**) for dynamic studies enable the objective evaluation and comparison of different approaches (**c.**).

means that a change in patient status can only be diagnosed with certainty if the measured value has changed by at least 80–100%. For a test which is expected to provide high sensitivity this is completely unacceptable. The reproducibility of the measurement procedure has to be improved and has to be assured by appropriate quality control procedures. In addition, the means for a comparison of results obtained with different scanners and scan modes have to be established.

In every respect, coronary calcium measurements therefore constitute a typical QCT application and have to be judged by the criteria defined above:

- Accuracy is not the most important criterium; however, appropriate calibration tools are required.

- Ensuring the highest possible reproducibility requires fixed scan protocols, dedicated reconstruction algorithms, automated evaluation procedures and calibration tools.

- For quality assurance a calibration standard should be measured at least as part of the monthly constancy testing, and preferably even along with each patient examination.

- Comparability of results obtained with different scanners is required to achieve general acceptance for the method. Here again, an established standard has to be developed and used.

Promising approaches for meeting these demands are available. Figure 7.6 shows a quality assurance phantoms and respective calibration inserts which have been developed at the IMP in collaboration with Siemens Medical Systems, the phantom manufacturer (QRM GmbH, Möhrendorf, Germany) and users of the SOMATOM Volume Zoom. For the present, this only represents a proposal. A consensus regarding calibration standards and quality assurance programs is urgently needed. This new field of application for CT is developing very rapidly. Long-term success will only be possible if the quality of the results, in particular reproducibility and comparability between different scanners, can be assured.

8   The Future of CT

The question of whether CT has a future at all was answered many times during the eighties – though incorrectly, as we now know. "CT is dead!" was a popular saying in view of the impressive developments which transpired in magnetic resonance tomography. And yet has CT lived on without complications and, in fact, during the nineties clearly experienced a renaissance. Today, CT is again undergoing a phase of rapid innovation.

We can examine the future of CT from several different points of view, from the clinical or the radiological point of view, from the economic point of view or from the standpoint of the physicist and engineer. For radiological diagnostics, the meaning of CT is determined largely in terms of daily routine. CT is fast and comfortable for the patient, with a high diagnostic reliability in its areas of application. Such innovations as multi-slice spiral CT represent further improvements, since MSCT simplifies and improves routine diagnostics. A good example is the acquisition of the complete lung during a single breath hold problem-free and with high and, to a good approximation, isotropic spatial resolution. The spatial resolution in all three dimensions is superior to that of competing modalities, and there are no geometric distortions.

The continued competitiveness and the particular capability of CT therefore derive from its proven and reliable simplicity, and not from as yet untapped potentials or promising new applications of immense complexity. CT applications are fast – in the meantime, a number of examinations can be completed in only a few seconds, that is comparable with a simple radiograph. Important for ensuring the simplicity of the method and good interpretability of the results is that the contrasts are clearly defined, with practically no dependence on the scanning parameters. Of course it is also necessary to recognize the disadvantage that a variety of contrast mechanisms, which is given for MRT, is not available for CT. In spite of this apparent limitation, however, the established diagnostic tasks of CT can be reliably clarified. This explains, for example, the pragmatically oriented development in recent years in the USA that cranial CT examinations have become one of the fastest growing radiological applications.

The economic efficiency of CT is also greatly superior to that of MRT and PET, as a direct comparison reveals. Equipment costs, just as in the computer field, have decreased much in spite of improvements in performance. For scanners of the highest performance class, prices in fact still lie typically between one and two million dollars, but scanners are now offered

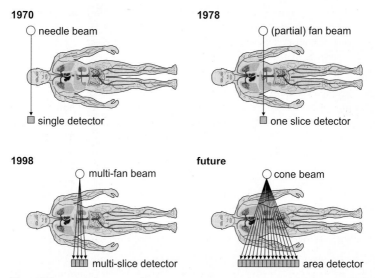

1970
○ needle beam

▣ single detector

1978
○ (partial) fan beam

▣ one slice detector

1998
○ multi-fan beam

▥ multi-slice detector

future
○ cone beam

▥ area detector

Figure 8.1
The development of CT from scanning with a pencil beam to scanning with a fan beam and multi-fan beams has already been fulfilled. The challenge for present and future developments is to make cone-beam CT available for clinical routine.

for less than 250,000 dollars as well, and – only ten years after the introduction of spiral CT – all scanners are now spiral-capable. An important development goal remains, however, fueled by the pressure of competition between different manufacturers, the reduction of costs.

Future developments in CT will also be defined by new fields of application. New applications can be expected in those disciplines where the high volume scan speed of MSCT now available can make important contributions: the heart, the lungs, in dynamic examinations and in CT angiography. Interventional procedures and computer-assisted surgery represent two other growth areas. New mobile CT scanners have also been developed for such applications.

Continuing technical developments in CT will sustain the trend already identified at the beginning of chapter 2: a higher speed of volume acquisition. This is made clear once again in figure 8.1. A further increase in the speed of rotation is fundamentally not excluded. More probable, however, appears to be the further development of detector technology, directed toward achieving finer arrays with a higher number of rows and greater variability in the selection of slice thickness and number of slices. While the problems entailed should not be underestimated, the trends are clearly set and there are no natural constants which could impose a rigid limit on the speed of rotation or the number of rows per detector array. Cone-beam

CT will certainly come; the question only remains, which cone angle (figure 2.12) is acceptable for which application. It is hardly necessary to mention further developments in regard to computer technology and therefore in performance capability for image reconstruction and display. These trends will positively affect CT and in fact all of radiology.

Cone-beam CT using area detectors and further improvements in spatial resolution in all three dimensions represent the decisive topics in research and development currently being pursued by many groups. Results are already available for the displays of high-contrast structures with high resolution, such as CT angiography with intra-arterial contrast medium injections or displays of bone microstructure (figure 2.12). The goal is to obtain high image quality with cone-beam geometry as well, especially the low-contrast resolution which has been available in clinical CT since its introduction. Higher spatial resolution is not the foremost goal for clinical CT, because this would require very high doses for structures with low contrast. The greater priority is to increase the rate of volume scanning further.

The future of CT will be decided not only by the assessment of its performance capability, but also by the dose values which CT acquisitions require. In earlier times, the performance capability was questioned, whereas today the "high dose" coupled with the recognized high performance capability is questioned. CT is evidently subject to observation and criticism in the eye of the public, even though such discussions generally focus on only a potential risk, but less so on the benefits of the method. Information on dose in CT is just as important as efforts to reduce dose. As already seen in chapter 5, it must be emphasized again that the classification as a "high dose procedure" is objectively not justified, since the effective dose for the patient is of the order of magnitude of the annual exposure to natural radiation. And, as shown in chapter 5, there is potential for a further reduction of patient dose.

My personal summary of the subject of CT: CT is alive and well, and it will live for many years to come. It represents a technically mature, low-risk method and can offer the patient very considerable benefits.

9 Appendix

9.1 Definitions

9.1.1 Abbreviations and Symbols

As far as possible, the following abbreviations and symbols conform with widely used standard definitions. To avoid defining new variables some symbols may occur with duplicate meanings. For example, the x-ray photon energy and the effective dose are both denoted by the symbol E. Due to the respective context it is assumed that confusions can be excluded.

2D	two-dimensional
3D	three-dimensional
a	sampling distance at the center of rotation in mm
a.p.	anterior-posterior
AEC	automatic exposure control
ART	algebraic reconstruction technique
ASSR	advanced single-slice rebinning
BERT	background equivalent radiation time
bpm	beats per minute
C	window center in Hounsfield units
CT	computed tomography
$CTDI$	CT dose index in mGy
D	number of detector rows
d	absorber thickness in cm
d	table feed per 360° rotation in mm
d'	table speed in mm/s
D_{FOM}	diameter of the field of measurement in cm
D_{FOV}	diameter of the field of view in cm
DLP	dose length product in Gy · cm
E	x-ray photon energy in keV

E	effective dose in mSv
EBCT	electron beam CT
ECG	electrocardiogram
FBP	filtered backprojection
FDA	Food and Drug Administration
FOM	field of measurement
FOV	field of view
$FWHM$	full width at half maximum in mm
$FWTA$	full width at tenth area in mm
$FWTM$	full width at one-tenth of maximum in mm
HU	Hounsfield unit
I	tube current in mA
I	x-ray intensity
I_o	primary intensity
$I(x,y,z)$	image function
I_i	value of pixel i
$\bar{I}$	mean pixel value of a region of interest
ICRP	International Commission on Radiological Protection
ICRU	International Commission on Radiation Units and Measurements
IMP	Institute of Medical Physics, University of Erlangen-Nürnberg, Germany
iMPR	interactive multiplanar reformation
LNT	linear no-threshold
M	number of simultaneously measured slices
MinIP	minimum intensity projection
MIP	maximum intensity projection
MPR	multiplanar reformation
MRT	magnetic resonance tomography
MSAD	multiple slice average dose
MCT	multi-slice CT

MSCT	multi-slice spiral CT
MTF	modulation transfer function
N_D	number of detector elements (channels) per detector row
N_{pixel}	number of pixels
N_{rot}	number of sequence scans or number of rotations
$O(x,y,z)$	object function
p	pitch factor
P	projection or attenuation value
P	power in W
p.a.	posterior-anterior
PET	positron emission tomography
pixel	acronym for picture element
pVR	perspective volume rendering
PSF	point spread function
Q	product of tube current and scan duration in mAs
QCT	quantitative CT
R	scan range in mm
R_D	radius of the detector center trajectory to the isocenter in mm
R_F	radius of the focal trajectory in mm
RI	reconstruction increment in mm
ROI	region of interest
S	slice thickness in mm
$S/d/RI$	common notation for spiral CT parameters: slice thickness / table feed per rotation / reconstruction increment
SI	scan increment of sequence scans in mm
SNR	signal-to-noise ratio
$SPQI$	slice profile quality index
SSCT	Single-slice spiral CT
SSP	slice sensitivity profile
STS	sliding thin slab
t_{rot}	time per 360° rotation in s

T	total scan time of a spiral scan in s
TLD	thermo-luminescence dosimetry
U	tube voltage in kV
UFC	ultra-fast ceramic
UNSCEAR	United Nations Scientific Committee on the Effects of Atomic Radiation
VE	virtual endoscopy
VOI	volume of interest
voxel	acronym for volume element
VR	volume rendering
w	interpolation weight
W	window width in HU
W	filter width
W_{D}	detector aperture in mm
W_{F}	focal spot size in mm
W_{pixel}	pixel size in mm
x,y,z	spatial coordinate system
z	z-position of the slice or the image
Z	atomic number
Z_{eff}	effective atomic number
ZF	zoom factor
α	view angle, projection angle or tube position in °
β	angle of a ray within the fan (x/y-plane) in °, $\beta_\in [-\varphi/2, \varphi/2]$
γ	angle of a ray within the cone (z-direction) in °, $\gamma_\in [-\kappa/2, \kappa/2]$
ε	total efficiency of the detector system
ε_{g}	geometric detector efficiency
φ	(full) fan angle in °
κ	(full) cone angle in z-direction in °
μ	linear attenuation coefficient in cm^{-1}
σ	standard deviation of pixel noise in HU

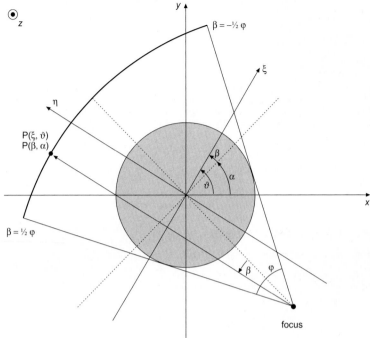

Figure 9.1
Definition of the coordinate system and of geometrical parameters describing the object sampling and image reconstruction in CT.

9.1.2   Geometry

Geometric parameters and relationships are briefly defined in chapter 1. In principle, a tomogram can be scanned in almost any arbitrary orientation. The typical orientation in CT and PET, however, is the so-called transverse or x/y-plane. The z-axis is perpendicular to the scan plane and to the image plane and thus parallel to the rotational axis of the gantry, and approximately parallel to the patient's longitudinal axis (figure 1.1). The sagittal plane thus corresponds to the y/z-plane and the coronal plane to the x/z-plane. Further important geometric parameters concerning the object sampling are illustrated in figure 9.1.

9.2   Mathematical Aspects of Image Reconstruction

9.2.1   Convolution

The so-called convolution integral $f * g$ of two functions f and g is of basic importance for signal processing in general and for image reconstruction in particular. The convolution results in a new function which is defined as follows:

$$h(x) = f(x) * g(x) = \int dt\, f(x-t)g(t).$$

Graphically this is the area below the function resulting when f is shifted by x and then multiplied by the function g.

In many applications, such as image processing and especially image reconstruction, the convolution is used for manipulating measured data. One of the two functions of the convolution integral plays the role of the measured data (e.g. $f(x)$), whereas the other function, called the convolution kernel or filter function, defines the manipulation of the measured data. The next section will show that the convolution of the measured attenuation profiles (projections) and the convolution kernel plays a decisive role for CT image reconstruction.

9.2.2 2D Radon Transformation

In two dimensions the Radon transform is the set of all possible line integrals of an object. Obviously, this corresponds directly to the measurement process in 2D CT. A line or pencil beam is defined by its signed distance to the origin and its angle with respect to the coordinate axes (figure 9.1). The projection data, i.e. the Radon transform, is given by integrating the object function along these lines. Using Dirać's delta function we can write:

$$p(\xi, \Theta) = \int d^2r\, f(r)\, \delta\, (r\Theta - \xi) \tag{9.1}$$

with $r = \begin{pmatrix} x \\ y \end{pmatrix}$ and $\Theta = \begin{pmatrix} \cos \vartheta \\ \sin \vartheta \end{pmatrix}$.

The task of image reconstruction is to invert this equation to solve for the unknown object function $f(r)$. A possible way to do so is to perform a 1D Fourier transform (denoted by the hat symbol) of the measured data $P(\xi, \Theta)$ with respect to ξ:

$$\hat{P}_l(u, \Theta) = \int d^2\xi\, P(\xi, \Theta)\, e^{-2\pi i u \xi}. \tag{9.2}$$

Substituting equation (9.1) into (9.2) will break the delta function down to yield

$$\hat{P}(u, \Theta) = \int d^2r\, f(r)e^{-2\pi i u r \Theta}. \tag{9.3}$$

It is then clear that the right-hand side is the 2D Fourier transform of the required object function, i.e.

$$\hat{f}(u\,\Theta) := \int d^2r\, f(r)e^{-2\pi i u r \Theta} \tag{9.4}$$

and we then arrive at what is known as the Fourier Slice theorem:

$$\hat{P}_l(u, \Theta) = \hat{f}(u\,\Theta),$$

the one-dimensional Fourier transform of the projections is the two-dimensional Fourier transform of the object function in polar coordinates.

A direct inversion of (9.5) using the inverse 2D Fourier transform to obtain $f(r)$ is in principle possible. This method, called Fourier- reconstruction, suffers from the problem of interpolating from the given polar grid $u\Theta$ (which is defined by the measurement process) to Cartesian coordinates u_i, i.e. interpolating from $\hat{f}(u\Theta)$ to $\hat{f}(u)$ ("gridding"). This method is prone to artifacts, since small scale interpolation errors in the Fourier domain will yield large scale errors in the spatial domain. Moreover, there is no natural way of incorporating reconstruction filters into the Fourier reconstruction that would allow us to modify the image quality (resolution, noise etc.).

Inverting the above equation without Fourier domain interpolations is therefore required. This can be obtained by an inverse 2D Fourier transform in polar coordinates $|u| \, du \, d\vartheta$ of equation (9.5) and by applying the convolution theorem for Fourier transforms:

$$f(r) = \int_0^\pi d\vartheta \int du \, |u| \, P_I(u, \Theta) \, e^{-2\pi i u r \Theta} = \int_0^\pi d\vartheta \, P(\xi, \Theta) * k(\xi) \Big|_{\xi = r\Theta} .$$

This reconstruction is called the filtered backprojection (FBP) algorithm. It consists of two steps: Convolution of the measured projection data $p(\xi, \Theta)$ for each view angle ϑ with the convolution kernel $k(\xi)$, followed by a backprojection of the convolved profiles $p(\xi, \Theta) * k(\xi)$ along the original beam direction $\xi = r\Theta$. The convolution kernel is taken to be the inverse Fourier transform of the ramp filter $\hat{k}(u) = |u|$. This obligatory convolution can be used in a natural way to add additional smoothing filters (mathematically known as an apodization or tapering function); typically a weight function $W(u)$ multiplies the ramp and $\hat{k}(u) = |u| \, W(u)$ is used for reconstruction. This has far-reaching consequences for the image quality since, as we can now see, the image quality can be influenced during the reconstruction process without additional computation. Examples are filters that accentuate high frequencies to improve spatial resolution (high resolution kernels), and kernels that attenuate high frequencies to reduce image noise and to improve low contrast resolution (smooth kernels).

Real measurements are discrete and the Radon transform is sampled at $\xi_i = \xi_0 + i\Delta\xi$. The convolution of the measured projections and the reconstruction kernel thus becomes the sum

$$p(\xi_i, \Theta) * k(\xi_i) = \sum_j p(\xi_{i-j}, \Theta) \, k(\xi_j).$$

The most famous and most important discrete reconstruction kernel is the Shepp-Logan kernel [Shepp, 1974]. Its representation is

$$k_j^{SL}(\xi_j) = \frac{2}{\Delta\xi^2 \pi^2 (1 - 4j^2)} .$$

The reason for the importance of the Shepp-Logan kernel is simply that it became available to the scientific community at an early stage through the publication of its analytical representation. Most kernels used in commercial CT scanners are treated as proprietary from the vendors and thus cannot be used by scientific groups for comparative studies.

9.2.3   3D Radon Transformation

In 3D the Radon transform is no longer the set of all possible line integrals (this would be called x-ray transform) but instead the set of all possible plane integrals of the object. These are integrals along planes defined by their distance to the origin and their normal vector Θ:

$$p(\xi, \Theta) = \int dr\, f(r)\, \delta\, (r\Theta - \xi)$$

$$\text{with } r = \begin{pmatrix} x \\ y \\ z \end{pmatrix} \text{ and } \Theta = \begin{pmatrix} \sin\theta \cos\vartheta \\ \sin\theta \sin\vartheta \\ \cos\theta \end{pmatrix}.$$

The inversion of the 3D Radon transformation can be obtained by exact analogy to the previous paragraph: either using direct Fourier inversion or using FBP. The generalization of the equations from 2D to 3D is straightforward since equations (9.1) through (9.5) remain valid after replacing d^2r by d^3r.

By contrast with the 2D case the Radon transform in 3D does not represent the measurement process. The reconstruction problem in 3D is to calculate (either explicitly or implicitly) the 3D Radon transform from the measured line integrals (3D x-ray transform). These line integrals correspond to rays emerging from the source at position heading in direction Θ:

$$p(s, \Theta) = \int d\lambda\, f(s + \lambda\Theta).$$

These line integrals could, in principle, be converted to plane integrals by adequate integration or by the summation of projection values. However, we are not dealing with a parallel geometry scan, and an integration of parallel line integrals to yield a plane integral is not possible. This is the main problem with the cone-beam reconstruction. There is so far no gold standard for cone-beam reconstruction, and numerous approaches can be found in the literature. In the following we will give a short survey of the most promising methods .

Cone-beam reconstruction algorithms can be divided into exact and approximate algorithms. The exact approaches try to convert the measured projection data (line integrals) into Radon data (plane integrals). The conversion formulas contain no approximations, since they are mathematically exact, hence the name "exact algorithms". This conversion can be either done by directly calculating the 3D Radon transform using the formula of Grangeat [Grangeat, 1991] or indirectly using a filtered backprojection approach [Defrise, 1994; Kudo, 1994]. Difficulties arise due to additional requirements. Either the complete object must be scanned ("long object problem") or special scan trajectories are required [Tam, 1998]. Initial approaches that try to fulfil most requirements for medical CT were recently published [Lauritsch, 2000]. Unfortunately they yield unacceptably long reconstruction times of several hours up to days for a typical scan volume.

The approximate algorithms introduce more or less severe approximations to invert the cone-beam data. Calculating the 3D Radon transform is strictly avoided. A typical procedure is to neglect the cone angle γ (the angle between the rays and the x/y-plane) or to consider only the increased path length by multiplying the projection values with cos γ. This helps to obtain 2D data which can be convolved with a reconstruction kernel similar to the 2D case. The final backprojection step then takes the 3D nature and the finite cone angle into account and a 3D backprojection is performed [Feldkamp, 1984; Yan, 1992; Schaller, 1997]. The resulting artifacts increase significantly with increasing cone angle, and most approximate reconstruction algorithms yield unacceptable results even for moderate cone angles.

A very promising method that assumes a spiral trajectory is the advanced single-slice rebinning (ASSR) [Kachelrieß, 2000a]. The spiral trajectory is approximated by a set of overlapping optimally tilted virtual 2D reconstruction planes. Rebinning is performed from spiral cone-beam data to the 180° parallel sequence data corresponding to these planes. These data can be reconstructed by using 2D FBP and the resulting tilted images are interpolated in the z-direction to yield Cartesian coordinates. ASSR, compared with other approximate cone-beam reconstruction algorithms, is the most promising method available today. The results are close to optimal for medical CT scanners with up to $M = 64$ simultaneously measured slices. Image quality, flexibility and computational requirements are adequate for use in future medical CT systems, where the expected increase in the number of simultaneously measured slices will force us to switch to cone-beam reconstruction algorithms.

10 Glossary

180° interpolation
a type of algorithm for → z-interpolation which utilizes a range of $2 \times 180°$ → projection angle within the measured → spiral CT data.

360° interpolation
a type of algorithm for → z-interpolation which utilizes a range of $2 \times 360°$ → projection angle within the measured → spiral CT data.

2D display
visual display of a 2D distribution, e.g. the reconstructed image of a CT scan displaying the distribution of the linear attenuation coefficient $\mu(x,y)$

3D display
visual display of a 3D distribution; since most display devices are 2D, various methods such as shading, movement or perspective are used to create a subjective 3D impression.

acceptance test
first test of the whole system after installation or after significant changes of the hard- or software; the acceptance test verifies the legal standards and the manufacturer's specifications; in addition the results of the acceptance test, as part of the → quality assurance, serve as a reference for the → constancy test measurements.

A/D conversion
abbreviation for → analog-to-digital conversion.

added filtration
thin metal sheets (commonly aluminum or copper) used for appropriate → filtration of the → x-ray spectrum emitted by the x-ray source in addition to the → intrinsic filtration.

air scan
→ sequential CT scan without object placed in the → gantry; the air scan is used to determine small differences in the individual → detector channel sensitivities and provides basic data for the → calibration of the CT system.

aliasing
results from violation of the requirements of the → sampling theorem; signal contributions with higher frequencies may affect the frequency range below the → Nyquist frequency in the form of → aliasing artifacts

aliasing artifact
artifact due to aliasing within the measured → projections; it appears in the reconstructed images as fine streaks and web-like patterns.

analog
term used in information theory to characterize a signal, e.g. the measured value of a physical quantity

which can adopt arbitrary values within a certain continuous range; for instance analog images provide an arbitrary fine gray scale and an infinitely high → geometrical resolution; see → digital.

Analog-to-digital conversion
conversion of an → analog input signal (a voltage in most cases) into a → digital output signal which can be processed by a digital computer.

anode
positive electrode, target of the → x-ray tube; the latter can be equipped with a stationary or with a → rotating anode.

anode angle
angle between the electron beam and a line orthogonal to the surface of the → x-ray tube's → anode.

anode load capacity
maximum permitted value of the instantaneous and of the mean long-term → x-ray tube power; the instantaneous maximum value for the tube current for a given tube voltage is determined by the melting point of the anode material and thus depends on the actual tube temperature, the size of the → focal spot and the duration of the electron beam impact on the → anode's surface; for short scan times such as with a single scan series or a single → spiral CT scan the permitted tube load depends mainly on the → x-ray tube's heat capacity; in the long run, i.e. for several series or over several hours, the tube capacity is limited by the rate of heat transfer from the → anode to the environment; see → rotating anode.

antiscatter grid
collimator system mounted in front of the → detector in order to remove → scattered radiation from the primary x-ray flux behind the object; the antiscatter grid is constructed of thin metal sheets aligned towards the → focal spot and almost completely absorbs those parts of the incoming radiation which do not originate from the focal spot.

artifact
part of the contents of an image that does not have a counterpart in the physical object being imaged; in CT images an artifact can appear as false structures (e.g. → aliasing artifact, → beam hardening artifact, → motion artifact, → partial volume artifact) or as a corruption of the → CT numbers.

attenuation
the decrease in the intensity of x-rays when passing through matter; the extent of attenuation is a property of the material which is exposed to radiation and is quantitatively described by the → linear attenuation coefficient; see → x-ray attenuation.

attenuation profile
spatial distribution of the total → x-ray attenuation of the object to be examined measured for a certain position of the x-ray source.

average CT value
arithmetic mean of the → CT numbers x_i of the pixels within a → region of interest:

$$\bar{x} = \frac{1}{n} \sum_{i=1}^{n} x_i \, ;$$

the mean → CT number for an object detail can be determined with high precision, although the single values are corrupted by → quantum noise.

axis of rotation
axis about which the CT apparatus (both the → x-ray tube and the → detector or the → x-ray tube alone) rotates during the measurement; see → direction of table feed, → z-axis.

backprojection
calculation of the contributions of each measured and filtered (see → convolution) → projection to the image to be reconstructed; the backprojection is the second step of the → filtered backprojection method for image reconstruction.

bar test pattern
physical phantom designed to measure the → spatial resolution; the bar test pattern can be realized by plastic bars embedded in a material with significantly lower contrast; with all bar test patterns for a specific set of identical bars the distance between the centers of the bars is always equal to twice the width of a single bar.

beam
the pack of primary → rays emerging from the → focal spot and contributing to the measurement of a single → attenuation value.

beam hardening
the change of the spectral distribution of → polychromatic radiation when passing through matter; since the photons with lower energy are absorbed with higher probability than those at higher energies, the mean energy of the → spectrum increases with the absorption length; the radiation becomes more penetrating ("harder"); in consequence the measured → x-ray attenuation per unit length for a specific material depends on the total thickness of the object.

beam hardening artifact
falsification of the structures of the imaged object or of the absolute CT numbers due to → beam hardening; beam hardening artifacts appear when the actual object differs significantly from the assumptions made by the → beam hardening correction with respect to the → x-ray attenuation; a critical region is e.g. the base of the skull.

beam hardening correction
preprocessing method to compensate for errors due to → beam hardening in the measured → projection data of a CT scan; the beam hardening correction is based on assumptions about the composition of a typical object to be scanned; see → dual-energy CT.

beam quality
distribution of the energy of → quanta forming an → x-ray beam; with an → x-ray tube the beam quality depends on the selected high voltage, the material of which the anode is made, the → anode angle and the presence of → additional filtration.

beam width
the width of the → x-ray beam within the → scan plane measured

in the direction orthogonal to the → beam's direction; the beam width is determined by the → scanner geometry, the → focal spot size and the → effective detector width.

bit
abbreviation of binary digit.

bit range
number of → bits used to store the value of a numerical entity; today CT numbers are stored typically with 12 bits, corresponding to the range of → Hounsfield Units from −1024 to +3071.

bore hole test pattern
physical phantom designed to measure the → geometrical or the → low-contrast resolution; the bore hole test pattern consists of a cylinder made of an appropriate material with sets of bore holes along the longitudinal axis of the cylinder and aligned in groups of holes with identical diameter and with a spacing of twice the hole diameter; with special bore hole test patterns the contrast can be varied by filling up the phantom with different liquids such that the → low-contrast resolution or → contrast-detail diagrams can be measured; also see → bar test pattern.

byte
unit cell for digital memory containing 8 → bits.

calibration
measurement for determining the individual → detector channel sensitivity for each → detector element of a CT system; the calibration is performed e.g. based on an → air scan and is applied during the → raw data pre-correction of data measured with an arbitrary object.

cardiac CT
see → cardiac imaging.

cardiac imaging
diagnostic imaging of a patient's beating heart; in order to avoid → motion artifacts and an unacceptable loss of → resolution the time for the measurement has to be extremely short (e.g. down to 100 ms with → electron beam CT) or the patient's → ECG has to be recorded simultaneously to the scan in order to perform prospective → ECG triggering (with → sequential CT scanning) or to enable retrospective → ECG-correlated image reconstruction (with → spiral CT scanning).

cathode
the negative electrode e.g. of a vacuum tube or an → x-ray tube.

central ray
→ ray emitted from the → focus and passing through the center of the exit window of the → x-ray tube that intersects the → axis of rotation.

ceramic detector
see → solid state detector.

ceramic scintillator
a ceramic material (e.g. Gd_2O_2S) with appropriate → doping (with e.g. Eu) such that light is emitted when exposed to radiation.

collimator
mechanical device for defining the shape of an → x-ray beam; every CT scanner is equipped with collimators between the → x-ray tube and the patient (pre-patient collimation) to define the → dose profile according to the requested → slice thickness; some machines additionally employ collimators between the patient and the → detector (post-patient collimation) for improving the → slice sensitivity profile by giving it a more rectangular shape; some machines have additional comb-shaped collimators close to the detector array to decrease the → effective detector element width and thus increase the achievable → geometrical resolution.

cone angle
aperture angle κ of a cone beam measured in the direction of the system → axis of rotation; also see → fan angle.

cone beam
pack of x-rays shaped like a cone, emerging from the → x-ray source → focus; see → fan beam, → ray.

cone-beam CT (CBCT)
CT system that is based on the measurements of → cone beam projections.

constancy test
physical performance test of a CT scanner, which has to be repeated at regular intervals (typically once per month); the constancy test is part of the → quality assurance and serves to verify that the system performance parameters are still identical with the initial performance

parameters at the time it was installed; see → acceptance test.

contrast
in CT commonly defined as the absolute difference between the → CT numbers of adjacent regions or structures within an image.

contrast detail diagram (CDD)
a diagram showing the minimum object contrast that is sufficient to resolve the bore holes in the image of a → bore hole test pattern for given scan parameters; the contrast is given as a function of the smallest visible bore hole diameter; a correct interpretation of a contrast detail diagram must be based on detailed information about the material and the size of the used test object, the selected → slice thickness, and the applied → dose, because these quantities directly influence the → pixel noise and thus significantly influence the contrast detail curve; see → low-contrast resolution.

contrast resolution
see → low-contrast resolution.

convolution
mathematical operation applied to two functions $f(x)$ and $k(x)$, where the latter is called the → convolution kernel; the result $g(x)$ is defined as
$$g(x) = f(x) * k(x) = \int f(t)\, k(x{-}t)\, dt$$
commonly the * symbol is used as an abbreviation for the convolution integral.

convolution kernel
in the connection with → image reconstruction for CT a special func-

tion used for → filtered backprojection, which can be varied within a certain range in order to tune the → pixel noise and the → geometrical resolution; see → convolution.

coordinate system
Cartesian $x/y/z$-coordinate system of the CT system; the scan plane is always the x/y-plane which is the → transverse plane in anatomy (except for non-zero → gantry tilt), the x-axis points in the lateral direction, the y-axis is oriented in the a.p. or p.a. direction; the → z-axis is orthogonal to the → scan plane; in most cases the x/z-plane and the y/z-plane are oriented parallel to the → coronal and → sagittal plane, respectively, in the anatomical sense.

coronal plane
anatomical plane orthogonal to the → transverse and the → sagittal plane; in the CT → coordinate system the coronal plane is usually oriented parallel to the x/z-plane.

crystal scintillator
a monolithic crystal (e.g. NaI) with appropriate → doping (with e.g. Tl) in which light is emitted when exposed to radiation.

CT dose index (CTDI)
ratio of the integrated → dose profile $D(z)$ (e.g. along the axis of rotation) and the total slice collimation $M \cdot S$; ideally the integration would range from – infinity to + infinity; in practice the range is 7 slice thicknesses ($CTDI_{FDA}$, defined by the FDA) or 5 cm ($CTDI_{100}$) on each side of the actual → slice plane; the $CTDI_{100}$ is calculated as

$$CTDI_{100} = \frac{1}{M \cdot S} \cdot \int_{-50 \text{ mm}}^{+50 \text{ mm}} D(z)dz.$$

frequently the CTDI is given normalized to a standard mAs product and weighted for different locations within the → scan plane (normalized weighted CTDI).

CT number
the final result of the CT measurement; the CT number is calculated from the → linear attenuation coefficient $\mu(x,y,z)$ reconstructed at a certain position in 3D space by scaling with the respective coefficient for pure water:

CT number $= \dfrac{\mu(x, y, z) - \mu_{water}}{\mu_{water}} \cdot 1000$ HU.

and is given in → Hounsfield Units (HU); see → x-ray attenuation.

CT value
synonymous with → CT number.

data acquisition system (DAS)
electronic subsystem of the CT apparatus, in which the detector output signals are amplified, integrated, multiplexed and → A/D converted.

density resolution
the CT system's capability to depict the small differences in the physical density of different human tissues; see → low-contrast resolution.

detector
in connection with CT a physical instrument to measure the intensity of incident x-rays; usually, CT scanners are equipped with → solid state detectors or → gas ionization detectors which both can provide high → x-ray absorption.

detector array
1D or 2D arrangement of the discrete detector elements.

detector channel
synonym for a single detector element.

detector channel sensitivity
the → sensitivity of a specific single → detector channel; the channel sensitivity is measured e.g. by an → air scan as a function of the detector channel number and is crucial for the → calibration of the scanner because due to slight variations in the detector manufacturing process (within the given tolerances) and small differences of the → x-ray absorption the individual → channel sensitivity varies and would lead to → ring artifacts without appropriate → raw data pre-correction.

detector element size
the cross section of a detector element orthogonal to the direction of the incident radiation has the shape of a rectangle; the length of the side of the rectangle which is parallel to the → scan plane determines the → effective detector width and in consequence the → beam width; the other side of the rectangle is usually oriented in the → z-direction and defines the maximum available → slice width.

detector quarter shift
the alignment of the → detector array for → fan beam systems in such a way that the → central ray strikes the → detector array with a shift of exactly one quarter of a single → detector spacing away from the contact zone between the two most → central detector channels of the → detector array (for an even number of detector channels, as is usual); the purpose of the detector quarter shift is to provide a shift of one half of the → detector spacing between opposing → projections (180° difference in → projection angle), thus allowing interlacing of opposing → projections and virtually doubling the → sampling frequency; this improves the → sampling and reduces → aliasing artifacts.

detector spacing
distance between the centers of two adjacent detector elements; the detector spacing in principle determines the → sampling distance for the measurement of a single → projection; see → sampling properties, → detector quarter shift.

digital
with discrete levels; discrete signals cannot adopt arbitrary values, but only a finite number of levels, depending on the number of → bits; see → analog.

direction of table feed
the direction of the table travel between successive sequential scans or during → spiral scanning; in most cases the direction of table feed coincides with the patient's longitudinal direction, and with the system's → z-axis (if no → gantry tilt is applied).

display window
freely selectable range within the → CT number scale displayed on the monitor screen and making use

of the full range of brightness levels of the display unit; usually the display window is defined according to its → window width and the → window center; all pixels of the → image matrix with a → CT number above the window center plus one half of the width are displayed as white, while those below the center minus one half of the window width are displayed as black.

doping
the contamination of a pure host material such as a crystal or a ceramic with small amounts of foreign atoms; if the base material is a → scintillator used in the construction of → x-ray detectors, appropriate doping can improve the → signal decay as well as the → absorption efficiency, or – in the best case – both.

dose
physical measure for the quantification of the energy released in matter due to exposure to radiation; see → effective dose, → energy dose, → equivalent dose,→ ion dose, → organ dose.

dose distribution
the spatial distribution of → dose as a function of the position within the → scan plane; the typical dose distribution in CT differs significantly from that in conventional radiography with respect to the decrease of dose from the surface towards the center of the object: in CT the ratio of the → surface dose and the dose at the center is in any case closer to one than for conventional radiography because the x-ray source rotates around the patient during the examination and thus there is radiation incident from nearly all directions.

dose efficiency
number that quantifies the amount of dose absorbed by the → detectors as a fraction of the total dose reaching the → detector; the dose efficiency is determined by the → geometrical dose efficiency and the → x-ray absorption of the detector material.

dose length product (DLP)
the product of the → x-ray tube current-time product C_i (in mAs), the normalized and weighted → CTDI value $_nCTDI_{100,w,i}$ (in mGy/mAs), the total → slice collimation $M_i \cdot S_i$ (in mm) and the number of rotations N_i added over all → sequential CT scan series or → spiral CT scans i:
$$DLP = \sum_i {}_nCTDI_{100,w,i} \cdot N_i \cdot M_i \cdot S_i \cdot C_i .$$

dose profile
the dose as a function of the position along the → axis of rotation resulting from a sequential scan; due to → x-ray scatter the dose profile is always broader than the → slice sensitivity profile, even if there is no post-patient (near to the detector) collimation.

dual-energy CT (DECT)
a method for scanning the same → slice successively with two different → x-ray spectra; by evaluation of the two measured attenuation values for the same → ray, specific physical properties of the material can be reconstructed, e.g. the electron density and the effective atomic number; dual-energy CT pro-

vides additional information that can be used e.g. to accurately determine the mineral content of bone, to perform a perfect → beam hardening correction, or to reconstruct images for a virtual → monochromatic x-ray source.

electrocardiogram (ECG)
recording of the bio-electrical signal of the heart muscles; the ECG allows for a detection of phases of slow (diastole, filling phase) and rapid (systole, ejection phase) motion of the heart and can be utilized for phase-selective imaging.

ECG-correlated image reconstruction
a method for → cardiac imaging, i.e. for retrospectively reconstructing spiral CT images for selected heart phases by correlating each measured → projection with the simultaneously recorded → ECG signal.

ECG triggering
prospective method for → cardiac imaging by triggering the CT scan on the basis of an → ECG signal that has to be evaluated in real time.

edge response function (ERF)
synonymous with → edge spread function.

edge spread function (ESF)
image of a high-contrast edge oriented orthogonal to the imaged plane; e.g. homogeneous objects made from PMMA within a water bath can be used in order to measure the ESF of a CT system if the object provides at least one even boundary plane oriented orthogonal to the → scan plane.

effective detector width
width of a single detector element within the → scan plane projected onto the → isocenter according to the → scanner geometry; see → detector element size.

effective dose
weighted sum of the mean → equivalent dose values H_T of single organs and tissues T; the normalized weights w_T describe the specific sensitivity to radiation → exposure of each organ or tissue as evaluated and published by the ICRP; the effective dose is defined as

$$E = \sum_T w_T \cdot H_T.$$

and has the unit Sv.

electron beam CT (EBT, EBCT)
alternative design of a CT scanner which functions without any moving mechanical parts; instead an electron beam is deflected and steered at high speed around the patient where the electrons hit an → anode ring and produce the fan of x-rays; while the concept is very attractive, it is now widely acknowledged that → spiral CT data acquisition with conventional → x-ray tubes is superior to EBT with respect to costs, image quality and range of possible applications.

electronic focal spot
area of intersection of the electron beam (produced at the → cathode) and the surface of the → anode of an → x-ray tube; see → focal spot.

electronic noise

contribution of the electronic devices of the → data acquisition system to the → projection noise of CT measurements.

energy dose

ratio of deposited energy per unit mass:

$$D = \frac{d\bar{\varepsilon}}{dm} = \frac{1}{\rho} \cdot \frac{d\bar{\varepsilon}}{dV}$$

where $d\bar{\varepsilon}$ is the mean energy deposited by ionizing radiation into a small volume dV of a material with mass dm and density ρ; the unit of energy dose is the Gray: 1 Gy = 1 J/kg.

entrance window

the front shield of a → detector on the side of the incident radiation; the entrance window is necessary for mechanical or electrical protection, but inevitably causes a decrease in the → dose efficiency of an → x-ray detector.

equivalent dose

defined as the weighted sum of the → energy doses D_R resulting from exposure to different kinds of radiation R (photon, neutron, α etc.); the equivalent dose H is calculated as

$$H = \sum_R w_R \cdot D_R$$

where w_R stands for the radiation quality weights; the unit is the Sievert: 1 Sv = 1 J/kg.

exposure

in connection with radiology the application of energy to the human body in the form of ionizing radiation (e.g. x-rays); due to the possibility of radiation damage following an exposure it is always necessary to consider the harms and the benefits prior to the application of ionizing radiation for the purpose of a radiological examination.

fan angle

angle α covered by the fan of x-rays within the → scan plane; see → field of measurement.

fan beam

x-ray beams that spread in fan-like geometry from an imaginary point-like → focus; the thickness of the fan beam is determined by the → collimators used to control the → slice width; see → fan angle, → cone beam, → ray.

fan-beam system

CT scanner for the measurement of each → attenuation profile of the object by means of a single fan of x-rays; thus, a single rotation of the x-ray source around the patient is sufficient to acquire a complete data set; there are two types of fan beam systems: so-called 3rd generation scanners, in which the → x-ray tube and a → detector arc rotate simultaneously and 4th generation scanners (→ ring detector), in which only the → x-ray tube rotates.

field of measurement (FOM)

region or volume for which complete data sets can be acquired; the size depends on the → scanner geometry and the → fan angle; the object to be scanned has to be within the FOM to avoid → artifacts due to data inconsistencies.

filtered backprojection

method for image reconstruction, which can be divided into two steps: → convolution and → back-projection of the measured → attenuation profiles; in principle the first step acts as a high-pass filter (enhancing of high signal frequencies) in order to avoid long-range smearing and degradation of details in the object image, which would occur when performing direct back-projection of the unconvolved → projections.

filtration
application of devices for → intrinsic filtration and → additional filtration between the → focus and the examined object; the filtration leads to a reduction of the lower-energy contribution of the → polychromatic x-ray spectrum; thus the radiation exposure of the patient is reduced without significant decrease of the measured signal, since these low-energy quanta are predominantly absorbed by the object and contribute little to the measured x-ray intensity; in addition the remaining x-ray distribution is less prone to → beam hardening, so that the → beam hardening correction is less complicated and → beam hardening artifacts are less frequent; see → form filter.

fluoroscopic CT
continuous imaging by CT to control or to guide a diagnostic or therapeutic intervention.

focus
idealized point on the surface of an → anode, at which the x-rays emerge; the focus is defined as the center of mass of the → electronic focal spot.

focal spot
region on the surface of the anode of an → x-ray tube, at which the incident electron beam produces x-rays; often the term focal spot is used synonymously with the → focus of the tube; see → electronic focal spot, → optical focal spot.

focal spot size
while the → electronic focal spot has a nonquadratic shape on the → anode surface (much larger in radial than in azimuthal direction) the tube is installed in the CT system in such a way that the → optical focal spot approximates a quadratic shape at the center of the detector array; for CT the focal spot size does not necessarily have to be small, since a finite → beam width due to an increased focal spot size is suitable for the suppression of → aliasing artifacts.

form filter
device for→ filtration of the x-ray beam; the thickness of form filters in CT increases with the distance from the → central ray, so that the difference in intensity measured at the detector between rays through the center of the object and peripheral rays, which experience low or no attenuation, is decreased; in addition by using form filters the intensity of → scattered radiation from peripheral parts and the patient dose are decreased; a perfect compensation for varying object thicknesses is not possible in principle because of the great differences in object shapes, which mostly deviate from a circular shape.

full-scan interpolation
sometimes used synonymous with → 360° interpolation.

full width at half maximum
distance on the abscissa of a 1D or 2D distribution between the points where the function reaches one half of its maximum value.

gantry
in CT the mechanical assembly including the → detector and the x-ray source, as the main part of the entire measurement system.

gantry tilt
tilt of the CT → gantry with respect to the patient by typically up to 30°; the → scan plane is rotated around the x-axis (→ coordinate system) such that the → axis of rotation and the → direction of table feed are not the same.

gas ionization detector
a → detector design for CT scanners, employing vessels filled with noble gas under high pressure; within the vessel the detector channels are separated by thin metal plates (→ septa) which are aligned towards the → focal spot of the → x-ray tube; each of the resulting cells acts as an ionization chamber connected to the → DAS via isolated transitions through the high pressure vessel for signal transfer.

geometrical dose efficiency
the amount of the radiation striking the → detector within the region in which the detector is sensitive to incident x-rays as a fraction of the total radiation dose leaving the patient; in practice the geometrical ef-

ficiency is below 100 % mainly due to postpatient → collimators and due to the inevitable presence of inactive areas between adjacent detector channels (→ septa); especially with → multi-row detectors the geometrical efficiency is an important parameter of the system; see → dose efficiency.

geometrical efficiency
synonymous with → geometrical dose efficiency.

geometrical resolution
the capability of a system to depict small structures of (arbitrarily) high contrast; the geometrical resolution can be quantitatively described by means of the → geometrical resolution limit, the → limiting spatial frequency, the → point spread function, the → edge spread function, the → line spread function and the → modulation transfer function.

geometrical resolution limit
resolution limit for (arbitrary) high contrast, expressed as the minimum size of an object detail that can be resolved.

half-scan interpolation
sometimes used synonymous with → 180° interpolation.

half width
sometimes used synonymous with→ full width at half maximum.

helical CT
synonymous with → spiral CT.

high-contrast resolution
synonymous with → geometrical resolution.

homogeneity
image quality parameter that describes the degree with which a test object made from a homogeneous material (e.g. a → water phantom) is depicted with constant → average value of the → CT number at varying positions within the image.

Hounsfield Unit (HU)
unit of the → CT number scale; the Hounsfield Unit expresses the relative deviation of the measured → linear attenuation coefficient from that of pure water, multiplied by 1000.

image archiving, compressed
recording of an → image matrix onto an arbitrary data medium by packing the information so as to achieve the maximum utilization of the data medium capacity; there are loss-less and lossy methods for compressed image archiving.

image archiving, uncompressed
recording of an → image matrix onto an arbitrary data medium without reducing the number of bits used to save each → pixel, keeping a fixed assignment of each single → pixel value to one data word.

image center
x/y-coordinates of the position at which the central point of the reconstructed image is located within the → scan plane; see → coordinate system.

image matrix
in CT the 2-dimensional arrangement of reconstructed values of the attenuation coefficient at discrete positions; the single elements are called → pixels.

image noise
noise contributions to the final image; see → pixel noise.

image reconstruction
calculation of the CT image from the → projection data.

image reconstruction algorithm
method used to reconstruct images from the measured → attenuation profiles; algebraic (iterative) algorithms that were used in the early stages of CT have been replaced by → filtered backprojection techniques in most cases today.

intrinsic filtration
filtration of x-ray beams due to the components of the x-ray source itself; the intrinsic beam filtration is caused for example by the anode itself, the glass of the vacuum vessel, the oil used for cooling and the x-ray exit window; a commonly used measure for the intrinsic beam filtration is the equivalent absorption length in aluminum; see → additional filtration.

ion dose
ratio of charge per unit mass:

$$I = \frac{dQ}{dm_{air}} = \frac{1}{\rho_{air}} \cdot \frac{dQ}{dV}$$

where dQ is the absolute amount of charge of one kind (positive or negative) produced directly or indirectly by ionizing radiation within a small volume dV of air; dm is the mass of air with density ρ_{air} within the volume dV; the unit of ion dose is C/kg.

isocenter
intersection of the → axis of rotation with the → scan plane.

Lambert-Beer law
→ x-ray attenuation.

limiting diameter
the diameter of the smallest holes of a → bore hole pattern which still appear separated in an image with given scan and reconstruction parameters; see → geometrical resolution limit.

limiting spatial frequency
the spatial frequency at which the modulation transfer function falls off to a certain minimum contrast which allows a sinusoidal → modulation of the given limiting spatial frequency yet to be determined; although the value of the minimum contrast is not commonly defined, the limiting value is often taken as 2 % of the zero frequency value of the → modulation transfer function; see → limiting diameter, → geometrical resolution limit.

linear attenuation coefficient
→ x-ray attenuation.

line response function (LRF)
synonymous with → line spread function.

line spread function (LSF)
image of an ideally infinitely thin plane oriented orthogonal to the → scan plane; the LSF of a CT scanner can be determined by measuring a thin plate oriented parallel to the → z-axis; in practice this

method is error prone and therefore replaced by measuring and differentiating the →edge spread function; see → point spread function.

low-contrast resolution
the geometrical → resolution for low-contrast details within the object; in addition to the → modulation transfer function of the CT system the → quantum noise and other sources of noise and artifacts inherent to the scanner determine the limit for separation of small low-contrast details within the image; see → contrast detail diagram.

matrix
2D arrangement of numbers; in the context of CT, used synonymously with the → image matrix.

matrix element
synonymous for picture element or → pixel.

measurement geometry
synonymous with → scanner geometry.

monochromatic radiation
x-ray beam with all its quanta having one and the same energy; see → polychromatic radiation.

modulation
a periodic variation of a signal in the spatial or temporal domain; the modulation is assumed to be a sinusoidal (→ modulation transfer function) or rectangular (→ square wave modulation transfer function) variation of the → attenuation when used to characterize the → spatial resolution in CT.

modulation transfer function (MTF, sinusoidal MTF)
the Fourier transform of the → point spread function; the MTF quantifies the relative contrast in the image of a sinusoidal → modulation as a function of the spatial frequency normalized to the zero frequency contrast; the MTF can be measured by scanning a thin wire (→ point spread function), an edge (→ edge spread function, → line spread function) or a → bar test pattern (→ square wave MTF).

motion artifact
artifact caused by movements of the object during data acquisition; the inconsistencies of the measured → projections not only result in unsharpness, as in conventional radiography, but can also cause long-range artifacts in the CT image.

multi-row detector
→ detector array with at least two, but typically between 4 and 64 independent detector rows; see → multi-slice system.

multi-slice system
CT scanner capable of measuring more than one slice simultaneously, based on → multi- row detectors or 2D → detector arrays.

multi-slice spiral CT (MSCT)
→ spiral CT scanning technique with the simultaneous acquisition of more than one independent slice; performed on → multi-slice systems.

noise
contributions to a measured signal due to random processes; in princi-
ple these contributions are of statistical nature and do not carry any information about the signal.

noise correlation
the relationship between two quantities that carry statistical → noise; for CT the reconstructed images show a noise correlation, i.e. the → pixel noise at one position within the image is not independent of that at other positions; the reason for this is the fact that with CT each measured → attenuation value contributes – although with significantly different weights – to every → pixel in the reconstructed image.

noise structure
non-regular patterns visible in a reconstructed CT image, caused by → noise and → noise correlation.

Nyquist frequency
spatial frequency that is determined by the → sampling distance a as:

$$u_{\text{Nyquist}} = \frac{1}{2a}$$

see → sampling theorem.

optical focal spot
projection of the → electronic focal spot parallel to the → central ray onto a plane orthogonal to the central ray.

organ dose
average dose applied over a complete organ within the body; the organ dose is required for the calculation of the → effective dose.

overscan
acquisition of more than 360° → projection angle range during a single slice scan; the additional data

range of about $10°$ to $40°$ is used to minimize inconsistencies which can occur between data acquired at the start and at the end of the scan, e.g. by averaging.

partial scan reconstruction
→ image reconstruction algorithm suitable for → fan beam scanners utilizing data from a projection angle range less than $360°$; the minimum data range is $180° + \varphi$ (see → fan angle φ); the partial scan reconstruction is used to enable shorter scan times in order to increase temporal resolution for → fluoroscopic CT or → cardiac CT.

partial volume artifact
artifact caused by severe inhomogeneities of the materials within the beam of the corresponding attenuation measurement (e.g. bone and air); the linear → attenuation coefficient μ as the physical quantity measured with CT depends on the attenuation length d, the incident intensity I_0 and the measured intensity behind the object I according to:

$$\mu \cdot d = \ln \frac{I_0}{I}$$

The averaging of the incident intensity within the detector element is not equivalent to an averaging of the attenuation coefficient itself; this is a source of nonlinear errors and thereby inconsistencies for attenuation measurements along different directions; partial volume artifacts occur within the slice (→ transverse plane) but especially in the → direction of table feed (increasingly with increasing → slice thickness).

phantom
object to test or evaluate the image quality of a CT scanner; there are → physical phantoms for real measurements and → virtual phantoms for mathematical simulation purposes.

phantom, homogeneous
→ phantom with spatially constant → x-ray absorption properties.

phantom, physical
object made of artificially made material, usually simulating the geometrical, → x-ray scatter and → x-ray absorption properties of biological objects; in addition there are physical phantoms with a mathematically defined shape for test purposes (e.g. → bar test pattern or → water phantom).

phantom, virtual
mathematical description of a virtual object as a basis for the simulation of CT data measurement; we can define abstract (e.g. spheres, boxes, etc.) or anthropomorphic virtual objects.

pitch
ratio of table feed per $360°$ rotation d and the total slice collimation $M \cdot S$:

$$p = \frac{d}{M \cdot S}$$

This definition is appropriate for single slice ($M = 1$) as well as for → multi-slice ($M > 1$) spiral CT. It is common practice to choose $1 \leq p \leq 2$; for cardiac CT, $p < 1$ is mostly required.

pixel
abbreviation of picture element.

pixel noise
statistical variation of the → CT number reconstructed for a single pixel within the → image matrix due to → projection noise within the measured → attenuation profiles; in the reconstructed image of an → homogeneous phantom or in homogenous parts of a → phantom the → pixel noise is seen as the statistical variation of the → CT numbers and is usually quantified with the → standard deviation evaluated for an appropriate → region of interest; the general validity of the pixel noise as a means to judge the image quality is restricted by the fact that the level of pixel noise depends on the → geometrical resolution via the → convolution kernel: pixel noise increases with increasing resolution.

point spread function (PSF)
the image of a line with infinitely small diameter oriented orthogonal to the image plane; in reality the PSF of a CT scanner can be measured by using a thin wire aligned parallel to the → z-axis; the wire's diameter has to be small compared with the expected → half width of the PSF; see → modulation transfer function (MTF).

polychromatic radiation
x-ray beam with a broad distribution (→ spectrum) of the energy of the emitted → quanta; the → x-ray tubes commonly used in diagnostic imaging produce polychromatic Bremsstrahlung; see → monochromatic radiation.

pre-correction
synonymous with → raw data pre-correction.

projection
in connection with CT, synonymous with the 1D or 2D → attenuation profile.

projection angle
angular position at which the x-ray source is located when measuring an → attenuation profile.

projection noise
→ noise within the → projections measured by a CT scan; the main sources for projection noise are → quantum noise and → electronic noise; today other sources of noise, such as the → A/D conversion or the discrete → image reconstruction algorithm can be assumed to be negligible.

quality assurance
see → acceptance test and → constancy test.

quantitative CT
clinical examinations with the purpose of quantitatively measuring geometrical, density, functional or other tissue or organ parameters; see → quantitative image evaluation.

quantitative image evaluation
based on digital images, e.g. CT images, various physical values can be quantitatively evaluated.

quantum
→ x-ray quantum.

quantum noise
noise contribution due to the random processes and the statistical nature of x-ray generation, → x-ray attenuation and x-ray detection; see → projection noise.

raw data pre-correction
preprocessing step that has to be applied to the measured "raw" → attenuation profiles in order to correct for the → beam hardening, the variation of the → sensitivity and the distance between single → detector channels, along with other sources of measurement errors; these corrections are inevitable and have to be performed before the actual → image reconstruction in order to achieve high image quality.

ray
idealized x-ray beam, having an infinitely small diameter.

reconstruction, reconstruction algorithm
synonyms for → image reconstruction algorithm.

reconstruction increment
the freely selectable spacing of images reconstructed from → spiral CT data sets along the → z-axis.

region of interest (ROI)
subset of pixels which lie within an arbitrary (circular, rectangular etc.) geometrical shape at a freely selectable position within a 2D image; based on this selection local statistical information can be calculated, e.g. the → standard deviation or the → average value of the → CT numbers.

resolution
see → geometrical resolution, → density resolution, → low-contrast resolution.

ring artifact
artifacts that appear as (partially) circular structures centered around the position of the → axis of rotation within the image; ring artifacts are caused by small differences of the → sensitivities between → detector channels for → fan beam systems with rotating detectors or by periodic variations of the x-ray intensity synchronously to the rotation and → data acquisition with → translation/rotation systems and → ring detector systems.

ring detector
→ fan beam scanner with the → detector elements positioned on a full circle and only the → x-ray tube rotating around the object; in most cases the detector ring is stationary and the x-ray source rotates inside the ring, but there have also been systems with the tube rotating outside of a detector ring nutating during the measurement, so that the detector elements close to the tube do not block the incident radiation.

rotating anode
an → x-ray tube → anode, shaped like a disc and kept in rotation around its own axis by an electric drive; the → focal spot is placed off-center, so that the position of the → focal spot on the disc surface changes continuously; a fixed volume of the → anode material is therefore exposed to radiation only transitorily and in consequence the temporary tube load can be significantly higher than that for stationary targets; because for rotating anodes the heat transport takes place mainly via dissipation of the thermal energy, these generally show a worse long-term load capability than → stationary anode

tubes with liquid cooling; see →
anode load capacity.

sagittal plane
anatomical plane oriented parallel
to the symmetry (median) plane of
the human body, orthogonal to the
→ transverse and the → coronal
plane; in the CT → coordinate
system the sagittal plane is usually
oriented parallel to the y/z-plane.

sampling, discrete
see → sampling distance.

sampling distance
distance between the equidistant
discrete points at which a continuous function is sampled for
measurement; see → sampling frequency.

sampling frequency
spatial frequency, expressed as the
reciprocal value of the → sampling
distance a:

$$u_s = \frac{1}{a}$$

sampling properties
ensemble of parameters which determine the sampling of the → projections during the CT scan; the
most important parameters are the
distance between single detector
channels (→ sampling distance),
the → detector quarter shift, the →
effective width of the detector elements and the angular increment
between successive projections.

sampling theorem
mathematical law, stating that a
continuous, band-limited function
can be completely recovered from
a finite number of measured values,

if this function does not contain
spatial frequencies above the →
Nyquist frequency; see → sampling
frequency, → aliasing.

scanner geometry
geometrical arrangement of the →
x-ray tube and the → detector with
respect to the → axis of rotation.

Scanogram
see → survey radiograph.

scan plane
the x/y-plane of the → coordinate
system; the scan plane contains the
focal trajectory and is consequently
the plane of rotation of the CT →
gantry; in most cases the scan plane
coincides with the → transverse
plane (see → gantry tilt).

scattered radiation
radiation emerging from an → x-
ray scatter process.

scintillator
substance that emits visible light
when exposed to radiation; used in
the construction of solid state detectors; see → ceramic scintillator,
→ crystal scintillator.

ScoutView
see → survey radiograph.

secondary reconstruction
image calculated from a series of
primarily reconstructed, adjacent or
overlapping CT images, having
nearly arbitrary orientation with respect to the → slice planes; usually
a secondary reconstruction is oriented orthogonal to the → slice plane;
see → sagittal plane, → coronal
plane.

semiconductor detector
x-ray detector made completely of a semi-conducting material; the incident radiation causes ionization within the material which is directly transformed into an electrical (current or voltage) output signal; see → solid state detector.

sensitivity
ratio of the magnitude of change of an output and the corresponding change of the input signal of an amplifier or → detector; see → detector channel sensitivity.

septa
thin metal plates separating adjacent ionization chambers of a → gas ionization detector: the septa are oriented parallel to the incident → x-rays and parallel to the → axis of rotation.

sequential CT
conventional CT scanning technique in which each requested slice is measured at a fixed z-position followed by an appropriate transport of the object in the → z-direction; for most applications today, the sequential CT technique has been replaced by → spiral CT.

sigma value
frequently used as synonym for → standard deviation.

signal decay
output signal of an x-ray → detector or an electronic amplifier as a function of time after the incident x-ray flux or the electrical input signal has been switched off; the signal decay of → detector systems

based on → scintillator materials can be improved by → doping.

Signal-to-noise ratio (SNR)
ratio of the intensity of a signal and the statistical fluctuation given by the corresponding → standard deviation.

slice plane
a plane oriented orthogonal to the → axis of rotation and located centrally within the slice of the object shown in the reconstructed image.

slice sensitivity profile (SSP)
the response measured in a CT image that results from an (ideally) infinitely thin object located on an axis parallel to the → z-axis as a function of the distance between the z-position of the scan and the center of the object; usually the SSP is normalized to one and depends on the radial distance of the axis to the → axis of rotation, i.e. on the location within the → field of measurement.

slice thickness
often used synonymously with → slice width.

slice width
in practice defined as the → full width at half maximum of the → slice sensitivity profile.

solid state detector
an → x-ray detector made of solid state materials; a solid state detector can be a pure semiconductor device or a → ceramic or → crystal scintillator in combination with a light sensitive semiconductor diode.

spatial frequency
reciprocal value of the wave length of a periodic structure in the spatial domain; spatial frequencies are given in units of cm^{-1}.

spatial resolution
in connection with CT, synonymous with spatial or → geometrical resolution; the spatial resolution has to be distinguished from the → density resolution and the → low-contrast resolution.

spectrum
in connection with → x-ray tubes, the distribution of energy levels of the quanta for → polychromatic radiation; see → beam quality.

spiral CT
method of CT scanning with continuous → gantry rotation and simultaneous continuous object translation in → z-direction; by contrast with the → sequential scan technique, with spiral CT the volume to be examined is sampled continuously along the → z-axis; during data acquisition the focus of the → x-ray tube follows a spiral trajectory relative to the object; the z-interpolation is introduced as an additional step during data preprocessing and allows a retrospective and arbitrary selection of the positions at which images are reconstructed.

square wave modulation transfer function (square wave MTF)
the relative contrast of the image of a rectangular → modulation as a function of the spatial frequency of the → modulation of the object with constant contrast; the square wave MTF can be evaluated directly from the scan of a → bar test pattern and can be used to calculate the sinusoidal → MTF; because the area below a half wave of a rectangular → modulation is larger than for a sinusoidal → modulation, the square wave MTF always yields better figures of merit when quantifying → spatial resolution; a comparison of two MTFs is therefore valid only if they are of the same kind.

square wave test pattern
synonymous with → bar test pattern.

standard deviation
statistical parameter for the quantification of the deviation of the single values from their → average value; if n is the number of samples x_i and $\bar{x}$ is the → average value, then the standard deviation is calculated as:

$$\sigma = \sqrt{\frac{1}{n-1} \cdot \sum_{i=1}^{n} (x_i - \bar{x})^2}$$

surface dose
amount of radiation dose that occurs at the body's surface.

survey radiograph
a projection image similar to a conventional radiograph measured with the CT scanner by moving the patient through the → gantry without gantry rotation; the survey radiograph is generated by displaying the → projections measured from a fixed → x-ray tube position for numerous table positions; by contrast with a conventional radiograph the digital survey radiograph in CT has

a cylindrical projection geometry; the various manufacturers denote this imaging modality e.g. as Topogram, Scout View or Scanogram.

system axis
synonymous with → axis of rotation.

system software
entirety of the various software tools forming part of the CT system, including the software for measurement control, → raw data pre-correction, → reconstruction, and display and evaluation of CT images.

Topogram
see → survey radiograph.

translation rotation system
CT scanner that performs a translation of the → detector and the → x-ray tube parallel to the → scan plane in order to linearly sample the → attenuation profiles; each translation is followed by a small rotational increment around the → axis of rotation to reach the next → projection angle.

transverse plane
anatomical plane orthogonal to the body's longitudinal axis; in connection with CT, in most cases identical with the → scan plane (except for non-zero gantry tilt); see → coordinate system.

water phantom
a commonly used → physical phantom for → quality assurance in CT; a water phantom is usually a PMMA cylinder filled with pure water or made from waterequivalent plastic.

voxel
synonym for volume element, for 2D CT images the voxel volume is defined by the width of the side of the → pixels and the → slice width.

window
synonymous with → display window.

window center
center of the → display window given in → Hounsfield units (HU).

window width
width of the → display window given in → Hounsfield units (HU).

xenon detector
→ gas ionization detector filled with the noble gas xenon at high pressure in order to achieve high → x-ray absorption.

x-ray absorption
basic physical ability of a material to absorb x-rays and transform their energy into other forms of energy, such as visible light, heat or fluorescence; in diagnostic imaging this process is dominated by Compton scatter and photoelectric absorption.

x-ray attenuation
the physical law which quantitatively describes the attenuation of the incident x-ray intensity I_0 when passing through a homogeneous object of thickness d and linear attenuation coefficient μ; μ depends on the energy of the → x-ray quan-

ta; the intensity of the radiation I measured behind the object can be calculated from $I = I_0 e^{-\mu d}$ (Lambert-Beer law); it should be mentioned here that this formula only holds for ideal conditions, i.e. in the absence of → x-ray scatter and for → monochromatic radiation, i.e. when all incident quanta have the same energy level.

x-ray beam
→ beam.

x-ray detector
→ detector.

x-ray quantum
smallest amount of energy carried by radiation and interacting with matter; the energy of the x-ray quantum is determined by the frequency ω or the wave length λ of the x-rays according to

$$E = \hbar\omega = \frac{hc}{\lambda}.$$

x-ray scatter: interaction process of x-rays with matter, changing the direction of the incident quanta only (Rayleigh coherent scatter) or both the direction and the energy (Compton incoherent scatter).

x-ray spectrum
→ spectrum.

x-ray tube
source of x-rays for nearly all CT systems; the x-ray tube consists of an → anode and a → cathode enclosed in an appropriate vacuum vessel; the spectral distribution and the intensity of the x-rays produced is controlled via the high voltage between the → anode and → ca-

thode and the tube current produced by the electrons leaving the cathode and striking the → anode.

x-ray tube power
electrical energy converted into heat and radiation per unit time; it is expressed as the product of the → x-ray tube voltage in kV and the tube current in mA; in practice the instantaneous maximum tube load determines the relationship between the maximum applicable dose for a given scan time respectively the maximum scan time for a given dose; the maximum long-term tube load determines the number of scans which can be performed on the average; see → anode load capacity.

z-*axis:* axis of the → coordinate system coinciding with the → axis of rotation.

z-*direction:* direction of the z-axis.

z-*interpolation:* a procedure for data preprocessing necessary before → image reconstruction from data measured with → spiral CT technique; the z-interpolation yields a data set representing a single planar slice by applying an interpolation method (usually linear); see → 180° interpolation, → 360° interpolation.

zoom factor
ratio of the diameter of the → field of measurement and the diameter of the volume shown in the image; together with the → image center the zoom factor determines which region of the object is reconstructed.

zoom reconstruction
→ image reconstruction with a large → zoom factor; the zoom reconstruction provides the magnification of regions within the image, similar to the magnification or lens tools; however, only the zoom reconstruction provides higher → geometrical resolution since it decreases the → pixel width.

11 References

Bauer, B.; Corbett, R.; Moores, B.M.; Schibilla, H.; Teunen, D. (Ed.): Reference doses and quality in medical imaging. Radiation Protection Dosimetry 1998; 80 (1–3)

Bielak, L.F.; Kaufmann, R.B.; Moll, P.P.; McCollough, C.H.; Schwartz, R.S.; Sheedy, P.F.: Small lesions in the heart indentified at electron beam CT: calcification or noise? Radiology 1994; 192: 631–636

Blank, M.; Kalender, W.A.: Medical volume exploration: gaining insights virtually. Eur. Radiol. 2000; 33 (3)

BMU (Bundesministerium für Umwelt, Naturschutz und Reaktorsicherheit): Umweltradioaktivität und Strahlenbelastung im Jahre 1996. Deutscher Bundestag 13. Wahlperiode. 1996; Drucksache 13/8630

Boyd, D.P.; Lipton, M.J.: Cardiac computed tomography. Proc. IEEE 1983; 71: 298–308

Bracewell, R.N.: Strip integration in radioastronomy. J. Phys. 1956; 9: 198–217

Bresler, Y.; Skrabacz, C.: Optimal interpolation in helical scan 3D-computerized tomography. National Science Foundation (MIP 88-10412) 1993: 1472–1475

Brooks, R.A.: Principles of computer assisted tomography (CAT) in radiographic and radioisotopic imaging. Phys. Med. Biol. 1976; 21: 689–732

Cameron, J.R.: A radiation unit for the public. Physics and society 1991; 20 (2)

Cohen, G.; Di Bianca, F.A.: The use of contrast-detail-dose evaluation of image quality in a computed tomography scanner. J. Comput. Assist. Tomogr. 1979; 3 (2): 189–195

Cormack, A.M.: Representation of a function by its line integrals, with some radiological applications. J. Appl. Physics 1963; 34: 2722–2727

Cormack, A.M.: 75 years of Radon transform. J. Comput. Assist. Tomogr. 1992; 16 (5): 673

Crawford, C.; King, K.: Computed tomography scanning with simultaneous patient translation. Med. Phys. 1990; 17: 967–982

Defrise, M.; Clack, R.: A cone-beam reconstruction algorithm using shift variant filtering and cone-beam backprojection. IEEE Trans. Med. Imag. 1994; MI-13: 186–195

Engelke, K.; Karolczak, M.; Lutz, A.; Seibert, U.; Schaller, S.; Kalender, W.A.: Mikro-CT. Technologie und Applikationen zur Erfassung von Knochenarchitektur. Der Radiologe 1999; 39 (3): 203–212

European Commission's Study Group (Ed.): Quality Criteria for Computed Tomography. EUR 16262. 1998

European Communities (Ed.): Council Directive 97/43/Euratom of 30 June 1997 on health protection of individuals against the dangers of ionising radiation in relation to medical exposure. Official Journal of the European Communities No. L 180/22 1997

Fahrig, R.; Fox, S.; Lownie, S.; Holdsworth, D.W.: Use of a C-arm system to generate true 3-D computed rotational angiograms. Am. J. Neuroradiology 1997; 18

Feinendegen, L.E.; Bond, V.P.; Sondhaus, C.A.; Altman, K.I.: Cellular signal adaptation with damage control at low dose versus the predominance of DNA damage at high doses. C.R. Acad.Sci., Science de la vie 1999; 322: 245–251

Feldkamp, L.A.; Davis, L.C.; Kress, J.W.: Practical cone-beam algorithm. J. Opt. Soc. Am. 1984; 1 (6): 612–619

Fellner, F.; Blank, M.; Fellner, C.; Böhm-Jurkovic, C.; Bautz, W.; Kalender, W.A.: Virtual Cisternoscopy of Intracranial Vessels: A novel Visualization Technique using Virtual Reality. Magnetic Resonance Imaging 1998; 16 (9): 1013–1022

Flohr, T.; Schaller, S.; Ohnesorg, B.M.; Klingenbeck-Regn, K.; Kopp, A.F.: Evaluation of image artifacts in multislice CT. Radiology 1999; 213(P): 317

Fuchs, T.; Kachelrieß, M.; Kalender, W.A.: Direct comparison of a xenon and a solid state CT detector system: measurements under working conditions. Physica Medica 1999a; XV (1): 48

Fuchs, T.; Krause, J.; Schaller, S.; Flohr, T.; Kalender, W.A.: Spiral interpolation algorithm for mult-slice spiral CT. Part II: Measurement and evaluation of slice sensitivity profiles and noise at a clinical multi-slice system. IEEE Transactions on Medical Imaging 2000; (in press) Special issue on Multislice CT.

Gies, M.; Kalender, W.A.; Wolf, H.; Süß, C.; Madsen, M.T.: Dose reduction in CT by anatomically adapted tube current modulation. I. Simulation studies. Med. Phys. 1999; 26 (11): 2235–2247

Grangeat, P.: Mathematical framework of cone-beam 3D-reconstruction algorithm for non-planar orbits. In: Mathematical Methods in Tomography. Lecture Notes in Mathematics. Berlin: Springer; 1991: 66–97

Greess, H.; Wolf, H.; Baum, U.; Kalender, W.A.; Bautz, W.: Dosisreduktion in der Computertomographie durch anatomieorientierte schwächungsbasierte Röhrenstrommodulation: Erste klinische Ergebnisse. Fortschr. Röntgenstr. 1999; 170 (1): 246–250

Hounsfield, G.N.: Computerized transverse axial scanning (tomography). Part I. Description of system. Br. J. Radiol. 1973; 46: 1016

Hu, H.: Multi-slice helical CT: Scan and reconstruction. Med. Phys. 1999; 26 (1): 5–18

ICRP: International Commission on Radiological Protection. Publication 60. Oxford: Pergamon Press, 1990

IEC: International Electrotechnical Commission: Medical electrical equipment – 60601 Part 2–44: Particular requirements for the safety of X-ray equipment for computed tomography. Geneva, Switzerland, 1999

Jawarowski, Z.: Radiation risk and ethics. Physics Today 1999; September: 24-29

Kachelrieß, M.: Reduktion von Metallartefakten in der Röntgen-Computer-Tomographie. Dissertation am Institut für Medizinische Physik, Universität Erlangen-Nürnberg, 1998a

Kachelrieß, M.; Kalender, W.A.: ECG-correlated image reconstruction from subsecond spiral CT scans of the heart. Med. Phys. 1998b; 25 (12): 2417–2431

Kachelrieß, M.; Kalender, W.A.: Dose reduction by generalized 3D-adaptive filtering for conventional and spiral single-, multirow and cone-beam CT: Theoretical considerations, simulations, phantom measurements and patient studies. Radiology 1999; 213(P): 283

Kachelrieß, M.; Schaller, S.; Kalender, W.: Advanced single-slice rebinning in cone-beam spiral CT. Med. Phys. 2000a; 27(4): 754–772

Kachelrieß, M.; Kalender, W.A.: ECG-correlated image reconstruction from subsecond multi-slice spiral CT scans of the heart. Med. Phys. 2000b; 27 (8): 1881–1902

Kalender, W.A.; Bautz, W.; Felsenberg, D.; Süß, C.; Klotz, E.: Materialselektive Bildgebung und Dichtemessung mit der Zwei-Spektren-Methode. I. Grundlagen und Methodik. Digitale Bilddiagn. 1987a; 7: 66-72

Kalender, W.A.; Hebel, R.; Ebersberger, J.: Reduction of CT artifacts caused by metallic implants. Radiology 1987b; 164: 576–577

Kalender, W.A.; Klotz, E.; Süß, C.: Vertebral bone mineral analysis: an integrated approach with CT. Radiology 1987c; 164: 419–423

Kalender, W.A.; Seissler, W.; Vock, P.: Single-breath-hold spiral volumetric CT by continuous patient translation and scanner rotation. Radiology 1989; 173(P): 414

Kalender, W.A.; Rienmüller, R.; Seissler, W.; Behr, J.; Welke, M.; Fichte, H.: Measurement of pulmonary parenchymal attenuation: use of spirometric gating with quantitative CT. Radiology 1990a; 175 (1): 265–268

Kalender, W.A.; Seissler, W.; Klotz, E.; Vock, P.: Spiral volumetric CT with single-breathhold technique, continuous transport, and continuous scanner rotation. Radiology 1990b; 176 (1): 181–183

Kalender, W.A.; Fichte, H.; Bautz, W.; Skalej, M.: Semi-automatic evaluation procedures for quantitative CT of the lung. J. Comput. Assist. Tomogr. 1991a; 15 (2): 248–255

Kalender, W.A.; Polacin, A.: Physical performance characteristics of spiral CT scanning. Med. Phys. 1991b; 18: 910–915

Kalender, W.A.; Polacin, A.; Eidloth, H.; Kashiwagi, S.; Yamashita, T.; Nakano, S.: Brain perfusion studies by xenon-enhanced CT using washin/washout study protocols. J. Comput. Assist. Tomogr. 1991c; 15 (5): 816–822

Kalender, W.A.: Spiral or helical CT: Right or wrong? Radiology 1994a; 193: 583

Kalender, W.A.; Polacin, A.; Süß, C.: A comparison of conventional and spiral CT: An experimental study on the detection of spherical lesions. J. Comp. Assist. Tomogr. 1994b; 18: 167–176

Kalender, W.A.: Principles and performance of spiral CT. In: L. W. Goldman and J. B. Fowlkes (Hrsg): Medical CT and Ultrasound: Current Technology and Applications. Madison, Wisconsin: Advanced Medical Publishing; 1995a: 379–410

Kalender, W.A.; Felsenberg, D.; Genant, H.K.; Fischer, M.; Dequeker, J.; Reeve, J.: The European Spine Phantom – a tool for standardization and quality control in spinal bone mineral measurements by DXA and QCT. Eur. J. Radiol. 1995b; 20: 83–92

Kalender, W.A.; Engelke, K.; Schaller, S.: Spiral CT: Medical Use and Potential Industrial Applications. Proceedings of SPIE. Developments in x-ray tomography 1997; 3149: 188–202

Kalender, W.A.; Schmidt, B.; Zankl, M.; Schmidt, M.: A PC program for estimating organ dose and effective dose values in computed tomography. Eur. Radiol. 1999a; 9: 555–562

Kalender, W.A.; Wolf H.; Süß, C.: Dose reduction in CT by anatomically adapted tube current modulation: II. Phantom measurements. Med. Phys. 1999b; 26 (11): 2248–2253

Kalender, W.A.; Wolf, H.; Süß, C.; Gies, M.; Greess, H.; Bautz, W.A.: Dose reduction in CT by on-line tube current control: principles and validation on phantoms and cadavers. Eur. Radiol. 1999c; 9: 323–328

Kaul, A.; Bauer, J.; Bernhardt, D.; Nosske, D.; Veit, R.: Effective doses to members of the public from the diagnostic application of the ionizing radiation in Germany. Eur. Radiol. 1997; 7: 1127–1132

König, M.; Klotz, E.; Luka, B.; Venderink, D.J.; Spittler, J.F.; Heuser, L.: Perfusions-CT of the brain: diagnostic approach for early detection of ischemic stroke. Radiology 1998; 209: 85–89

Kopka, L.; Funke, M.; Breiter, N.; Hermann, K-P.; Vosshenrich, R.; Grabbe, E.: Anatomisch adaptierte Variation des Röhrenstroms bei der CT. Untersuchungen zur Strahlendosisreduktion und Bildqualität. Fortschr. Röntgenstr. 1995a; 163 (5): 383–387

Kopka, L.; Funke, M.; Fischer, U.; Vosshenrich, R.; Oestmann, J.W.; Grabbe, E.: Parenchymal Liver Enhancement with Bolus-triggered Helical CT: Preliminary Clinical Results. Radiology 1995b; 195: 282–284

Kudo, H.; Saito, T.: Derivation and implementation of a cone-beam reconstruction algorithm for non-planar orbits. IEEE Trans. Med. Imag. 1994; MI-13: 186–195

Lauritsch, G.; Tam, K.C.; Sourbelle, K.; Schaller, S.: Exact local regions-of-interest in spiral cone-beam filtered-backprojection CT: numerical implementation and first image results. SPIE Medical Imaging Conference 2000; ME 3979–50

Luckey, T.D.: Physiological benefits from low levels of ionization radiation. Health Physics 1982; 43 (6): 771–789

Matanoski, G.M.: Health effects of low-level radiation in shipyard workers. Final report. Baltimore, MD. 1991

McCollough, C.H.; Zink, F.E.: Performance evaluation of a multi-slice CT system. Med. Phys. 1999; 26 (11): 2223–2230

McFarland, E.G.; Brink, J.A.; Loh, J.; Wang, G.; Argiro, V.; Balfe, D.M. et al.: Visualization of colorectal polyps with spiral CT colography: evaluation of processing parameters with perspective volume rendering. Radiology 1997; 205: 701–707

Miles, K.; Dawson, P.; Blomley, M. (Ed.): Functional Computed Tomography. Oxford: Isis Medical Media 1997

Mori, I.: Computerized tomographic apparatus utilizing a radiation source. United States Patent Number Dec. 16 1986; 4630202

Morneburg, H. (Ed.): Bildgebende Systeme für die medizinische Diagnostik. München: Publicis-MCD 1995

Mossman, K.L.: The linear no-threshold debate: Where do we go from here? Med. Phys. 1998; 25 (3): 279–284

Ohnesorge, B.; Flohr, T.; Schwarz, K.; Heiken, J.P.; Bae, K.T.: Efficient correction for CT image artifacts caused by objects extending outside the scan field. Med. Phys. 2000; 27(1): 39–46

Parker, D.L.: Optimal short scan convolution reconstruction for fanbeam CT. Med. Phys. 1982; 9 (2): 254–257

Polacin, A.; Kalender, W.A.; Marchal, G.: Evaluation of section sensitivity profiles and image noise in spiral CT. Radiology 1992; 185 (1): 29–35

Polacin, A.; Kalender, W.A.; Brink, J.A.; Vannier, M.: Measurement of slice sensitivity profiles in spiral CT. Med. Phys. 1994; 21: 133–140

Radon, J.H.: Über die Bestimmung von Funktionen durch ihre Integralwerte längs gewisser Mannigfaltigkeiten. Ber. vor Sächs. Akad. Wiss. 1917; 69: 262–277 (english translation available: J. Radon: On determination of functions from their integral values along certain manifolds. IEEE Transactions on Medical Imaging 1986; MI-5(4): 170–176)

Ritchie, C.J.; Godwin, J.D.; Crawford, C.R.; Stanford, W.; Anno, H.; Kim, Y.: Minimum scan speeds for suppression of motion artifacts in CT. Radiology 1992; 185 (1): 37–42

Robb, R.; Hoffmann, E.; Sinak, L.J.; Harris, L.D.; Ritman, E.L.: High-speed three-dimensional x-ray computed tomography: The dynamic spatial reconstructor. Proc. IEEE 1983; 71: 308-319

Rossmann, K.: Point spread-function, line spread function, and modulation transfer function. Radiology 1969; 93: 257–272

Rothenberg, L.; Pentlow, K.S.: CT dosimetry and radiation safety. Advanced Medical Publishing. Madison, Wisconsin. Medical CT & Ultrasound. Current Technology and Applications. 1995: 519–556

Royal College of Radiologists: Making the best use of department of clinical radiology: guidelines for doctors. 4th edition, London: Royal College of Radiologists. 1998

Rubin, G.D.; Beaulieu, C.F.; Argiro, V.; Ringl, H.; Norbash, A.M.; Feller, J.F. et al.: Perspective volume rendering of CT and MR images: applications for endoscopic imaging. Radiology 1996; 199: 323–330

Schaller, S.; Flohr, T.; Steffen, P.: New, efficient fourier-reconstruction method for approximate image reconstruction in spiral cone-beam CT at small cone- angles. SPIE Medical Imaging Conference Proc. 1997; 3032: 213–224

Schaller, S.; Flohr, T.; Klingenbeck, K.; Krause, J.; Fuchs, T.; Kalender, W.A.: Spiral interpolation algorithm for multi-slice spiral CT. Part I: Theory. IEEE Transactions on Medical Imaging 2000; (in press) Special issue on Multislice CT.

Scudder, H.J.: Introduction to computer aided tomography. Proceedings of the IEEE 1978; 66 (6): 628–637

Shepp, L.A.; Logan, B.F.: The fourier reconstruction of a head section. IEEE Trans. on Nuclear Science 1974; NS-21: 21–43

Shope, T.B.; Gagne, R.M.; Johnson, G.C.: A method for describing the doses delivered by transmission x-ray computed tomography. Med. Phys. 1981; 8: 488–495

Shrimpton, P.C.; Jones, D.G.; Hillier, M.C.; Wall, B.F.; Le Heron, J.C.; Faulkner, K.: Survey of CT Practice in the UK; Part 2: Dosimetric Aspects. Oxon: National Radiological Protection Board – R 249, 1991

Simmons, J.A.; Watt, D.E.: Radiation protection dosimetry: a radical reappraisal. Madison, Wisconsin: Medical Physics Publishing, 1999

Süß, C.; Kalender, W.A.: Performance evaluation and quality control in Spiral CT. In: L. W. Goldman and J. B. Fowlkes (Hrsg): Medical CT and Ultrasound. Madison, Wisconsin: Advanced Medical Publishing; 1995: 467–485

Süß, C.; Kalender, W.A.; Coman, J.M.: New low-contrast resolution phantoms for Computed Tomography. Med. Phys. 1999; 26 (2): 296–302

Taguchi, K.; Aradate, H.: Algorithm for image reconstruction in multi-slice helical CT. Med. Phys. 1998; 25 (4): 550

Tam, K.C.; Samasekera, S.; Sauer, F.: Region-of-interest cone beam CT with a spiral scan. SPIE Medical Imaging 1998; 3336: 274–283

Toki, Y.: Principles of helical scanning. In: K. Kimura and S. Koga (Hrsg): Basic principles and clinical applications of helical scan: Application of continuous-rotation CT. Tokyo: Iryokagakusha; 1993: 110–120

Toth, T.; Crawford, C.; King, K.: Moving beam helical scanning. Radiology 1991; 181(P): 278

Ulzheimer, S.; Kachelrieß, M.; Kalender, W.A.: New phantoms for quality assurance in cardiac CT. Radiology 1999; 213(P): 402

UNSCEAR: United Nations Scientific Committee on the Effects of Atomic Radiation 1994. Report to the General Assembly, with Scientific Annexes. United Nations Publications, 1994

Vining, D.J.; Liu, K.; Choplin, R.H.; Haponik, E.F.: Virtual bronchoscopy: relationships of virtual reality endobronchial simulations to actual bronchoscopic findings. Chest 1996; 109: 549–553

Vock, P.; Jung, H.; Kalender, W.A.: Single-breathhold spiral volumetric CT of the lung. Radiology 1989; 173(P): 400

Yan, X.; Leahy, R.M.: Cone-beam tomography with circular, elliptical and spiral orbits. Phys. Med. Biol. 1992; 37: 493–506

Zankl, M.; Panzer, W.; Drexler, G.: The calculation of dose from external photon exposures using reference human phantoms and Monte Carlo methods. Part VI: Organ doses from tomographic examinations. Neuherberg, 1991

Index Terms